Healthy Habits FOR

Your Heart

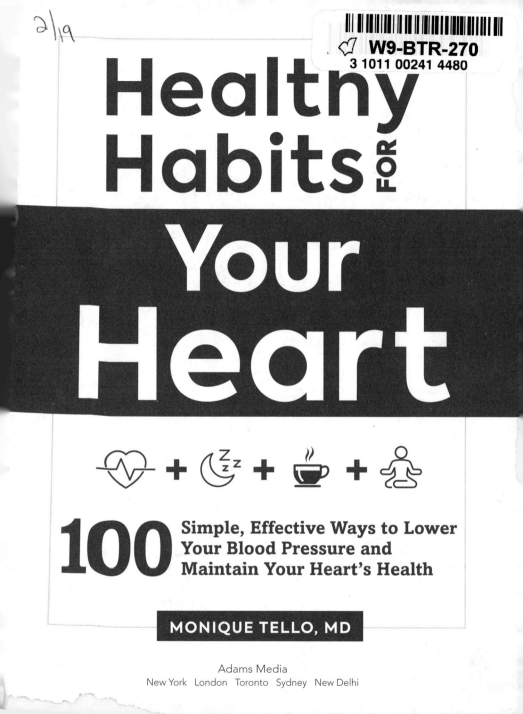

100 Simple, Effective Ways to Lower Your Blood Pressure and Maintain Your Heart's Health

MONIQUE TELLO, MD

Adams Media
New York London Toronto Sydney New Delhi

▲adamsmedia

Adams Media
An Imprint of Simon & Schuster, Inc.
57 Littlefield Street
Avon, Massachusetts 02322

First Adams Media trade paperback edition December 2018

ADAMS MEDIA and colophon are trademarks of Simon & Schuster.

For information about special discounts for bulk purchases, please contact Simon & Schuster Special Sales at 1-866-506-1949 or business@simonandschuster.com.

The Simon & Schuster Speakers Bureau can bring authors to your live event. For more information or to book an event contact the Simon & Schuster Speakers Bureau at 1-866-248-3049 or visit our website at www.simonspeakers.com.

Interior design by Michelle Kelly
Interior images by Dave Forbes

Manufactured in the United States of America

10 9 8 7 6 5 4 3 2 1

Library of Congress Cataloging-in-Publication Data
Tello, Monique (Medical doctor), author.
Healthy habits for your heart / Monique Tello, MD.
Avon, Massachusetts: Adams Media, 2018.
Series: Healthy habits.
Includes index.
LCCN 2018037078 (print) | LCCN 2018037739 (ebook) | ISBN 9781507209240 (pb) | ISBN 9781507209257 (ebook)

Subjects: LCSH: Heart--Diseases--Prevention. | Heart--Diseases--Diet therapy. | Physical fitness. | BISAC: HEALTH & FITNESS / Diseases / Heart. | HEALTH & FITNESS / Diseases / General. | COOKING / Health & Healing / Heart.
Classification: LCC RC682 (ebook) | LCC RC682 .T45 2018 (print) | DDC 616.1/205--dc23
LC record available at https://lccn.loc.gov/2018037078

ISBN 978-1-5072-0924-0
ISBN 978-1-5072-0925-7 (ebook)

DEDICATION

To the people without whom I could never have written this book: My best friend and life partner, Bob Socci: When I got this contract, I turned to you and said, "Honey, this is MY Super Bowl." You let me take the ball and run with it. My mom, Nancy Tello: Neither Bob nor I nor the kids could do anything without you. You're super-Nana, because you help everyone else find their wings and fly. My kids, Maria and Gio: You're both so, so little, but you "got" how important this project was to me right away. My dad, Jorge E. Tello, and brother, Jorge F. Tello: As physician colleagues you inspire me, as family members you support me, and I am deeply appreciative. I love you all.

ACKNOWLEDGMENTS

Thanks to my friends and colleagues who provided their knowledge, experience, and time to better inform this book. In alphabetical order:

- Fatima Cody Stanford, MD, MPH, MPA: Obesity Medicine Physician Scientist at Massachusetts General Hospital and Harvard Medical School
- Linda Delahanty, MS, RD, LDN: Director of Nutrition and Behavioral Research, Massachusetts General Hospital Diabetes Center; Assistant Professor of Medicine, Harvard Medical School
- Stephanie Eisenstat, MD: Internist, Massachusetts General Hospital; Assistant Professor of Medicine, Harvard Medical School
- Cassidy Salus, Chef de Cuisine: Boston-Area Farm-to-Table and Pastry
- Anne Thorndike, MD, MPH: Internist, Cardiovascular Disease Prevention Center, Massachusetts General Hospital; Assistant Professor of Medicine, Harvard Medical School
- Kathleen Ulman, PhD, CGP, DFAGPA: Psychologist, Massachusetts General Hospital; Assistant Professor of Psychiatry (Psychology), Harvard Medical School
- Deborah Wexler, MD, MSc: Clinical Director, Massachusetts General Hospital Diabetes Center; Associate Professor of Medicine, Harvard Medical School
- Malissa Wood, MD, FACC, FASE: Codirector, Corrigan Women's Heart Health Program, Massachusetts General Hospital; Associate Professor of Medicine, Harvard Medical School

And, of course, special thanks to all of my patients who graciously shared their experiences and insights. Though they cannot be named, they are what this book is all about.

CONTENTS

INTRODUCTION

Your heart's the most important organ in your body. You might not think about it much, but hour after hour, day after day, year after year it's pumping blood through your arteries, carrying oxygen and vital nutrients to your organs, and keeping you alive.

But your heart is vulnerable. Heart disease is the number one cause of premature death in the United States and the world. The good news is that most cases are preventable, simply by adopting small, everyday healthy habits. Forming the healthy habits that protect your heart is safe, effective, and inexpensive. When you put enough of these habits in place, you will transform your whole lifestyle, and you will:

- Lose weight and keep it off
- Prevent, manage, and even cure high blood pressure, high cholesterol, and diabetes
- Prevent heart disease and related medical problems, such as strokes

It's true—healthy lifestyle changes can be as effective as prescription medications, and without the costs and side effects. Breaking old bad habits and establishing new healthy ones is possible! This book shows you how to create your own safe, healthy, realistic lifestyle-change program. You'll learn about the heart and heart disease and how the risk factors for heart disease can be impacted by your lifestyle choices. You'll learn why you may want to make changes and how you can make those changes last. You'll see the evidence behind specific recommendations and how to break it all down into everyday habits. You will learn simple and straight-forward ways to:

- Manage stress and relax
- Sleep longer and better
- Form and improve relationships
- Enjoy healthy food
- Move more, more easily
- Live smarter

And more. In this book, there are 100 habits that will keep your heart—and the rest of your body, for that matter—healthy and happy.

Note: All of my current patients provided written permission to be interviewed specifically for this book. Names and any identifying details have been changed.

PART 1

Heart and Habit Basics

Chapter 1: Heart Science will explain why the heart is so incredibly important to your body and how it works. You'll learn what heart disease is, what the risk factors are, and how all of them can be prevented or managed.

Chapter 2: Your Heart Is in Your Hands will cover how heart disease can be prevented and even cured by a healthy lifestyle. You'll see how healthy lifestyle change can be achieved through targeting your everyday habits.

Chapter 3: How to Change Your Habits will reveal the science of habit and the psychology of behavior change, as well as many techniques you can use to help make your healthy lifestyle habits stick.

Chapter 1

Heart Science

DOCTORS WISH THEY HAD MORE TIME with you to explain things. You or someone you care about may have heart concerns, and there are questions you'd like answered. In this chapter you'll learn why heart disease is such a major issue; how the heart works; and about heart and related diseases, including explanations of medical terms. Finally, you'll learn what the risk factors are and how they are impacted by diet and lifestyle habits.

Heart Disease Is a Huge Problem

Heart disease is officially the number one cause of death in the world, accounting for 31 percent of all deaths. In the United States, heart disease is the number one cause of death for both men and women, accounting for one in every four deaths. It's the most common cause of premature death, and countless years of productive and fulfilling life are lost due to heart disease every day.

Heart disease is often a stealthy killer. According to government statistics, about half of sudden cardiac deaths happen outside of a hospital. Because heart disease can be silent for years, and symptoms can be different in different people, many don't recognize they even have heart disease until it's too late.

But what is heart disease, how does it happen, and what are the risk factors? First let's learn why the heart is such an important organ.

What Your Heart Does

Your heart is the constantly running engine of your circulation, pumping oxygen-heavy red blood cells to all of your organs and pulling used-up blood full of carbon dioxide away from them. The blood never stops moving, flowing in an endless continuous loop.

If we had to choose a starting place, we could start where bright red oxygen-heavy blood from the lungs is pumped out of the left side of your heart and into your arteries. Your arteries pulse, contracting in time with your heart, pushing blood and oxygen all over your body. As the oxygen is used up, the old bluish blood is pulled through your veins back to the right side of your heart, which pushes that old blood through your lungs. When you breathe in, you refresh all those blood cells with oxygen, the bluish blood turns bright red, and the cycle starts again.

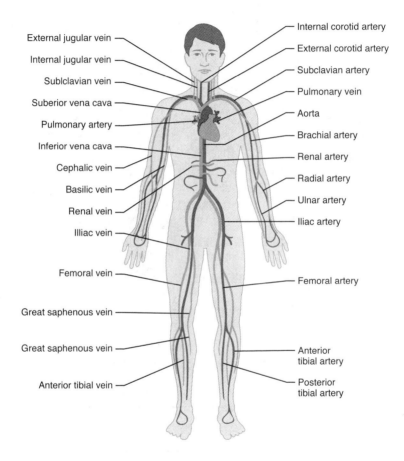

External jugular vein

Internal jugular vein

Sublclavian vein

Suberior vena cava

Pulmonary artery

Inferior vena cava

Cephalic vein

Basilic vein

Renal vein

Illiac vein

Femoral vein

Great saphenous vein

Great saphenous vein

Anterior tibial vein

Internal corotid artery

External corotid artery

Subclavian artery

Pulmonary vein

Aorta

Brachial artery

Renal artery

Radial artery

Ulnar artery

Iliac artery

Femoral artery

Anterior
tibial artery

Posterior
tibial artery

The circulatory system

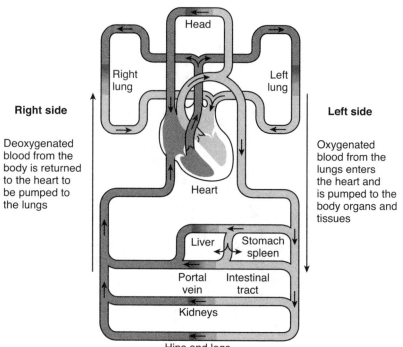

The circulatory system is a continuous loop.

Your heart and blood vessels are all connected. Blood from the right side of the heart flows through the lungs to the left side of the heart, and blood from the left side of the heart flows through the entire body and back to the right side of the heart. It's all one big life-giving loop.

How Your Heart Does It

Your heart is a fist-sized organ made of hardworking muscle, and like any other organ in your body, it needs oxygen. The arteries that feed the heart have to be wide open in order to deliver oxygen-heavy red blood cells to that working muscle.

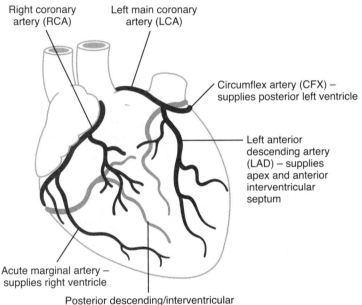

Right coronary artery (RCA)

Left main coronary artery (LCA)

Circumflex artery (CFX) – supplies posterior left ventricle

Left anterior descending artery (LAD) – supplies apex and anterior interventricular septum

Acute marginal artery – supplies right ventricle

Posterior descending/interventricular artery (PD) – supplies posterior septum

The coronary arteries descend down and wrap around the heart like a crown over a head, hence the name. *Crown* is *corona* in Latin and *kornē* in Greek.

Your heart never rests. Every minute it contracts—or beats—an average of seventy times and pumps about 5½ liters of blood. When you exercise, your heart can pump 20 liters of blood per minute. Over an entire day, it beats about one hundred thousand times.

Every heartbeat is sparked by tiny regular electrical currents. It's these electrical currents that appear on an electrocardiogram, or ECG. During an ECG, each of the twelve sticky leads that is stuck to the patient's body "sees" the electrical current from a different angle:

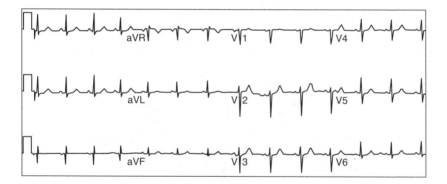

This is a normal, reassuring ECG.

If the arteries that feed the heart become blocked, the heart muscle can become sick or damaged, which will interfere with the electrical impulses. That's why an abnormal ECG can be a sign of heart disease.

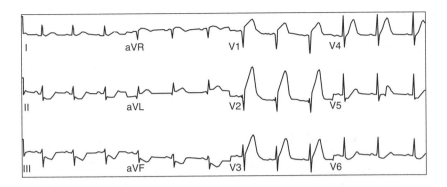

This is an abnormal ECG showing a heart attack in progress.

What Is Heart Disease?

The term *heart disease* can refer to a bunch of similar medical problems. Most are caused by the same things and commonly coexist.

Coronary Heart Disease

When we refer to heart disease, we're usually talking about coronary heart disease. In the medical chart, this may be abbreviated as CHD (or CAD, short for coronary artery disease, which is the same thing). In coronary heart disease, cholesterol and calcium deposits form plaque in our arteries. When plaque builds up, blood can't flow through very well. The blood can then clot up what little space was left, and the artery can become completely blocked, which can cause chest pain and heart attacks.

Atherosclerosis

The fancy term for plaque buildup in the arteries is *atherosclerosis*, also called "hardening of the arteries." Plaque can build up in any artery. We commonly see this in the aorta, your largest artery, which arches up from your heart and then runs all the way down your chest and abdomen, as well as the carotids, which run up either side of your neck to your brain.

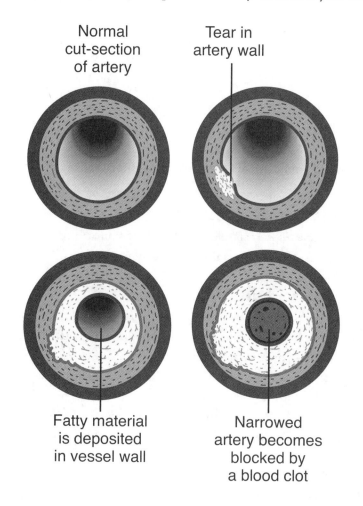

Normal cut-section of artery

Tear in artery wall

Fatty material is deposited in vessel wall

Narrowed artery becomes blocked by a blood clot

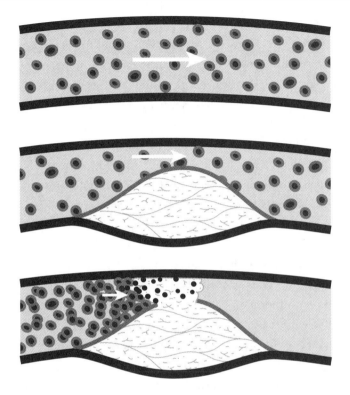

These images show normal and progressively worsening atherosclerosis. It's important to know that this process can occur in any artery.

While genetics can play a part in this process, the biggest cause by far is the way we eat and live. Poor diet, inactivity, stress, and sleep problems can lead to high blood pressure, which damages the delicate lining of the insides of the arteries. Being overweight and obese can lead to high cholesterol and abnormal blood sugars, which help form plaque.

Microvascular Disease

When we think of arteries, we usually think of the big muscular ones like the aorta and carotid arteries or the critically important coronary arteries. But there is a vast network of tiny arteries that also is essential for our bodies to function well—especially our heart and brain. All things that cause plaque in the larger arteries can cause plaque in the tiny ones, and this is called *microvascular disease*. People with uncontrolled diabetes, especially women, are at particularly high risk for microvascular disease. This is what causes the eye, nerve, and kidney complications in diabetes (called *diabetic retinopathy*, *neuropathy*, and *nephropathy*).

Angina

Classically, coronary heart disease causes chest pain, and that pain is called *angina*. If there's a lot of plaque buildup in an artery of the heart, it can become almost completely blocked. When a person is calm and at rest, she may not have any idea that there's a serious problem. When she gets stressed or exerts herself, her heart beats faster and harder. That blockage can prevent blood from getting to the heart muscle, so it becomes starved of oxygen, and that usually hurts. The pain can be in the chest, jaw, neck, or shoulder. However, angina is not always painful and may only be experienced as shortness of breath, nausea, heartburn, or other symptoms that come on with exertion and get better with rest.

Case Study:
Angina Isn't Always Painful

"I struggled to get here from the parking garage," huffed the wiry older man.

I was working in an urgent care clinic, and I had never met this patient before. I looked through his chart and saw that he had coronary heart disease. His case was thought to be mild, and he knew this. "My wife made me come in," he explained. But his medical history and symptoms raised red flags. We arranged for a stress test, but he could not finish the test. He could not catch his breath, and the technician saw worrisome ECG changes. Off he went to the emergency room, where he was shown to have a significant blockage in his left main coronary artery, the one referred to as *the widowmaker*. He was lucky his wife had made him come in. The lesson: any unpleasant symptoms brought on by activity and relieved by rest could be angina.

Complications of Coronary Heart Disease

If left untreated, coronary heart disease can lead to heart attacks and heart failure. It's important to know that diet and lifestyle changes alone can cure coronary heart disease, and these measures plus medications are even more powerful.

Heart Attack

A thick-enough plaque (atherosclerosis) and clotted blood can cause an artery to become clogged. This starves the heart of oxygen, and if the blocking plaque is not cleared, the muscle will die and the heart will be damaged. This is a heart attack, though you may see it on a medical record as a myocardial infarction (MI). When the heart muscle is damaged, it can scar, and the heart cannot function correctly. This can then lead to heart failure and even strokes.

What's Bad for the Heart Is Bad for the Head

The tiny arteries of the heart can get blocked with plaque, causing chest pain and heart attacks. This is called *microvascular disease*, and it's also a big problem in the brain. Microvascular disease in the brain can cause dementia, called *vascular dementia*. It's also a big contributor in Alzheimer's disease. Research shows that people who live unhealthy lifestyles are far more likely to also have dementia, and if they already have Alzheimer's, they'll have a worse case.

Of course the opposite is also true—a healthy lifestyle protects against dementia, even Alzheimer's. It's the number one thing patients who have a family history of Alzheimer's and want to protect their brain should adopt: a healthy diet, regular activity, good self-care.

Heart Failure

When the heart muscle is damaged, from whatever cause, it can't pump very well. This is called *cardiomyopathy*. When the heart can't pump well, blood and fluid get backed up in the lungs. This is congestive heart failure, or CHF for short. A person with CHF will have leg swelling and shortness of breath, which can become life-threatening. The most common cause of CHF is heart muscle damage from heart attacks, but there are other causes as well.

Other Forms of Heart Disease

There are other forms of heart disease, and it's important to know about them.

Coronary Heart Disease Without Obstructed Arteries

We've mentioned how some people don't have the usual symptoms with their coronary heart disease. It's also true that some people (particularly women) don't have the usual form of coronary heart disease. As a matter of fact, people can even have a heart attack without having any significant coronary heart disease. If a person is showing evidence of a heart attack by symptoms, ECG changes, labs, and/or imaging, but there are no significant blockages found on a coronary artery catheterization, it's still a heart attack, and an underlying cause must be found. There is a new medical term for when this happens, and it's *myocardial infarction with nonobstructive coronary arteries*, or MINOCA for short.

The possible causes of MINOCA include spasms of the arteries of the heart, called *coronary artery vasospasm*; plaque in the tiny arteries of the heart, called *microvascular disease*; ripping of the inner layer of the coronary arteries, called *spontaneous coronary artery dissection* (SCAD for short); and stress-induced heart failure, also called *the broken heart syndrome*. These are all far more common in women, and only recently are they being more carefully studied.

Arrhythmia

An irregular heartbeat is called an *arrhythmia*. This can be deadly on its own or can also cause strokes. There are different kinds, some brought on by heart attacks.

The most common arrhythmia by far is atrial fibrillation, also known as Afib. The irregular heartbeat of Afib can cause irregular blood flow in the left atrium of the heart, similar to the swirling eddies along the edges of a stream. Irregularly flowing blood can clot, and those clots can go flying up the aorta and into the arteries leading to the brain, causing strokes. This is why people with Afib take blood thinners, which help prevent clots.

A common cause of Afib is long-standing high blood pressure. Over time, as the heart has to pump against a high pressure, it can become distorted. For this reason the risk of Afib is especially high in people with a history of poorly controlled high blood pressure.

Diseases Related to Coronary Heart Disease

The same things that cause coronary heart disease can also cause other serious circulatory problems.

Aortic Aneurysm

We've already mentioned the aorta, the largest artery in the body. High blood pressure, smoking, and plaque buildup can cause a swelling to form in the aorta, called an *aortic aneurysm*. When an aortic aneurysm gets too large, surgery may be required or it can burst and be deadly.

People with a family history of these are at higher risk, as well as people over sixty, and especially men.

Peripheral Arterial Disease

There are many arteries in the body, and when plaque affects the arteries of the legs, it's called *peripheral arterial disease* (PAD). This can result in pain while walking, which can be disabling. Sometimes surgery is necessary, but regular physical activity can help a great deal.

Strokes

Strokes kill 6.7 million people worldwide every year and injure or disable millions more. Some strokes are caused by bits of blood clot that form in the heart and then travel through the arteries to the brain, where they can block blood supply and cause brain damage. Both heart failure and irregular heartbeat can cause those blood clots to form. Strokes are also called *cerebrovascular disease*. Strokes are commonly caused by unhealthy lifestyles, and people with strokes often also have coronary heart disease and other arterial diseases.

Are You at Risk for Heart Disease?

You've learned how the heart works and all about heart and related diseases. But what are the risk factors? Science has shown us what factors increase risk for heart disease, and these include genes, certain diseases, and lifestyle factors. Here's the key takeaway message though: even if you have genetic or disease risk factors, lifestyle choices can greatly impact your chances of developing heart disease. (As we'll learn in Chapter 2, healthy lifestyle choices can even reverse heart disease in someone who already has it!) Nothing is written in stone, and anyone can lower their risk.

Genetic Factors

These are risk factors that we are born with.

Family History

When a patient has a family history of coronary heart disease, or related diseases like strokes and aortic aneurysms, doctors need to listen and get details. We especially want to know about parents and siblings, and how old they were when they first had these problems. If you had a father or a brother with heart disease before age fifty-five, or a mother or a sister with heart disease before age sixty-five, that puts you at higher risk.

While you may be genetically predisposed to conditions and diseases that lead to heart disease—high blood pressure, high cholesterol, diabetes—it's very important to know that the way you eat and live can prevent and reverse those conditions and diseases.

Race/Ethnicity

African Americans tend to be more salt-sensitive, which may explain why they have a higher risk of high blood pressure that's difficult to control. They are also at greater risk for obesity and diabetes than Caucasians. Native Americans, Latinos, and certain Asian ethnic groups are also at higher risk for obesity, diabetes, and metabolic syndrome—all diseases that are associated with heart disease.

It's again important to note that a healthy lifestyle can help everyone avoid the diseases that are associated with heart disease. But unlike pure genetics, race and ethnicity factors can be more complicated. Research shows that racial and ethnic minorities don't always receive the medical treatment that they need and tend to have more complications and deaths from heart disease. Studies suggest that this is due to social, political, and economic differences that result in unequal access to care. This inequality is a massive problem and is an area of active research.

Gender

Heart disease, not breast cancer, is the number one leading cause of death in women. But many women, approximately one out of nine women in fact, will be diagnosed with breast cancer at some point, and they have to worry about both. One reason is that heart disease and breast cancer have some of the same risk factors, including obesity and smoking. Another is that some breast cancer treatments can be toxic to the heart, such as certain chemotherapies, and definitely radiation therapy. Women are surviving longer after a diagnosis of breast cancer, which is a good thing, but they should be informed about their increased risk for heart disease and receive the appropriate nutrition and lifestyle counseling. This is because, again, healthy choices can still lower their risk of heart disease.

Disease Factors

Certain medical conditions are associated with increased risk of heart and related diseases. Most of these medical conditions can be prevented or reversed with diet and lifestyle adjustments, and possibly other treatments.

High Blood Pressure

There is a definite, indisputable association between high blood pressure and heart disease. High blood pressure affects the heart and circulation in several ways. Sheer stress on the smooth lining of the arteries causes damage, making it easier for plaque to build up. This not only contributes to coronary heart disease but also to strokes and peripheral arterial disease. That high pressure can also cause distortion and ballooning of arteries, called *aneurysms*. These can burst and be deadly. Not only that, but when the pressure in the arteries is high, the heart has to pump harder to push blood around the body. Over time as the heart works harder, it can get distorted, with some areas of thickening and other areas of bulging. This can lead to irregular heartbeat and even heart failure.

A 20-point higher than normal systolic blood pressure or a 10-point higher than normal diastolic blood pressure doubles the risk of death from heart disease or related diseases (like stroke and abdominal aortic aneurysm). The good news is that a healthy diet (especially a plant-based, low-salt diet, which we'll talk more about in Chapter 5), regular physical activity, and stress management have all been proven to help lower blood pressure. Simply changing what you eat can bring down systolic blood pressure by as much as 11 points, and each additional healthy habit you adopt can bring it down another 4 to 5 points. Per the updated guidelines, these holistic strategies are now first-line approaches in many cases of high blood pressure.

What's High Blood Pressure?

High blood pressure is called *hypertension*. Blood pressure is measured in millimeters of mercury (mm Hg). The top number is the systolic, and the bottom number is the diastolic. The 2017 guidelines tell us:

- Normal blood pressure = under 120/80
- Elevated blood pressure (not yet hypertension) = systolic between 120 and 129
- Stage 1 high blood pressure (hypertension) = systolic between 130 and 139 or diastolic between 80 and 89
- Stage 2 high blood pressure (more severe hypertension) = systolic over 140 or diastolic over 90

High Cholesterol

When you get your labs report from your doctor, you see a bunch of different types of cholesterol listed: total cholesterol, high-density lipoprotein (HDL or "good" cholesterol), low-density lipoprotein (LDL or "bad" cholesterol"), and triglycerides. The LDL, or bad cholesterol, is particularly associated with plaque and atherosclerosis, the cause of most coronary heart disease.

Doctors can also use a formula (from the American College of Cardiology) to determine who has a risk of 10 percent or more of developing heart disease within the next ten years. The formula takes into account age, sex, race, blood pressure, total cholesterol, HDL and LDL levels, and if they are already taking an aspirin or medicine for high blood pressure or high cholesterol.

What's a High Cholesterol Level?

The following ideal LDL levels vary based on a person's risk factors.
- LDL under 160 mg/dl: for people with zero or one risk factor
- LDL under 130 mg/dl: for people with two or more risk factors
- LDL under 100 mg/dl: for people who already have heart or a related disease

The main risk factors are:
- Smoking
- Age (men over age 45, women over age 55)
- High blood pressure
- Diabetes
- Family history of heart disease
- Low HDL (under 40 mg/dl)

Diet and lifestyle recommendations are the first-line treatment for high cholesterol. Certain fats, such as trans fats and saturated fats, are associated with heart disease, through toxic effects on the blood vessels. But what really pushes our body to make loads of bad cholesterol is regularly eating sugars and refined grains (like white flour), being physically inactive, and/or being obese. Having a family history can certainly contribute, and there are rare diseases that can cause dangerously high cholesterol. Therefore, it is strongly recommended that people at risk eat a healthy diet, be as physically active as possible, and get to a healthy body weight. It is also recommended that certain people who are at particularly high risk start a cholesterol-lowering medication, like a statin.

High Blood Sugar (Diabetes)

When we talk about high blood sugar and heart disease, we're usually talking about type 2 diabetes. But it's important to understand: type 1 (juvenile) and type 2 (adult-onset) diabetes are both major risk factors for heart and related diseases. Both involve insulin, the hormone that allows sugar to enter the cells of the body. But while type 1 is caused by not enough insulin, type 2 is caused by too much.

Insulin is made in the pancreas. In type 1 diabetes, the pancreas stops making insulin altogether, causing sugar to build up to dangerous levels in the bloodstream. The cells of the body "starve," which sets off a dangerous metabolic cascade called *ketoacidosis*. Without insulin injections, type 1 diabetes is fatal. We don't know why some people develop type 1 diabetes.

Diet and lifestyle can cause type 2 diabetes. People with a family history of type 2 diabetes or who had gestational diabetes (diabetes in pregnancy) are at especially high risk. A diet high in sugars and refined carbohydrates (sugary drinks, sweets, and refined flours like white flour) can trigger surges of insulin. Over time the cells become resistant to all the insulin surges, which is called *insulin resistance*. Regularly eating meat (particularly red meat) also contributes to insulin resistance, perhaps through a toxic effect of heme iron, which is only found in animal meats. The pancreas makes more and more insulin, trying to overcome the resistance, but eventually it gives out. This leaves high blood sugar levels hanging around in the bloodstream, which is type 2 diabetes. Sugar sticks to the lining of the arteries, especially where damage and plaque are. This speeds up the process of atherosclerosis, causing blockages in the arteries of the heart and all over the body. People who have diabetes are at higher risk for heart and related diseases, as well as complications and death from those diseases.

How Do You Measure High Blood Sugar?

There are two main ways to measure blood sugar:

1. The fasting blood sugar is drawn after an 8-hour fast and is measured in milligrams per deciliter (mg/dl). This test is very reliable and inexpensive.

   Fasting blood sugar under 100 = normal
   Fasting blood sugar 101–125 = prediabetes
   Fasting blood sugar over 126 = diabetes

2. The hemoglobin A1c (HbA1c for short) can be drawn anytime. The HbA1c measures the percentage of sugar stuck to the red blood cells, which circulate around the body for three months; therefore, the HbA1c estimates the average blood sugar over three months.

   HbA1c under 5.6 percent = normal
   HbA1c 5.7 percent–6.4 percent = prediabetes
   HbA1c over 6.5 percent = diabetes

Type 2 diabetes is not only a major cause of heart and related diseases; it also is the leading cause of kidney failure, blindness, and amputations. Diet, lifestyle changes, and weight loss are very effective for preventing and treating type 2 diabetes, even for people with prediabetes who are at especially high risk. In a large study of more than one thousand adults with prediabetes, a diet, lifestyle, and weight loss program followed for 24 months lowered the risk of diabetes by 58 percent after three years, 34 percent after ten years, and 27 percent after fifteen years, without any medications. This approach, called the Diabetes Prevention Program, was so effective that, as of 2018, insurance companies are willing to pay for this intensive diet and lifestyle change program for people who are at risk for diabetes.

Obesity

Being obese increases risk of high blood pressure, high cholesterol, high blood sugars, and metabolic syndrome significantly. Obesity is also in and of itself associated with increased risk for an early death.

Many of us tend to gain weight in middle age, which can be dangerous: in a study of more than one hundred thousand people followed for several decades, even 11 pounds of weight gain toward middle age was associated with significantly higher rates of type 2 diabetes, cardiovascular disease (including heart disease), and cancer.

The flip side of this is that even a modest amount of weight loss can decrease these risks. An analysis of fifty-four studies showed that weight loss interventions for people with obesity decreased their risk of premature death, and especially death from cardiovascular disease (including heart disease), significantly. Losing even just 9 to 15 pounds has been shown to lower the risk of developing diabetes by 33 percent. In the very successful Diabetes Prevention Program described earlier, the ideal goal for weight loss was 7 percent of total body weight, which for a 225-pound person is about 15 pounds.

Overweight and Obesity: How Are These Calculated?

We use the body mass index (BMI) to calculate if someone is a healthy weight. The easiest way to know your BMI is to Google "BMI calculator" and plug in your height and weight. The manual way is: divide your weight in pounds by your height in inches squared; then multiply the result by a conversion factor of 703.

The formula is BMI = weight in pounds/[height in inches × height in inches] × 703

- Underweight = BMI under 18.5
- Healthy Weight = BMI 18.6–24.9
- Overweight = BMI 25–29.9
- Obese = BMI 30–39.9
- Morbidly Obese = BMI 40 and up

The BMI takes into account weight and height, but not muscle mass, so athletes with dense muscle mass may have a high BMI, even though they're healthy. Likewise, people with very low muscle mass, like many elderly folks, may have a normal BMI, but because they are weak and carrying a disproportionate amount of fat, they are at greater risk for many negative health outcomes. This is called *sarcopenic obesity*, and doctors have proposed lowering the definition of obesity in elderly people to a BMI of 28. However, for most people, the BMI works fine.

Metabolic Syndrome

Metabolic syndrome means having three or more of the following:

- Abdominal obesity (waist circumference more than 35 inches in women, 40 in men)
- High fasting blood sugars (over 100 mg/dl)
- Abnormal cholesterol (triglycerides over 150 or HDL under 40)
- High blood pressure (over 130/85)

Having three or more of these conditions is associated with about double the risk of developing type 2 diabetes, heart disease, and related diseases, like strokes, and a greater risk of complications or death from those diseases. The good news? People can avoid or reverse metabolic syndrome through healthy diet, physical activity, and weight loss.

Inflammatory Diseases

Any disease that causes inflammation in the body can increase the risk of heart disease. Evidence suggests that inflammation promotes damage to blood vessels and contributes to atherosclerosis. Rheumatoid arthritis is definitely linked to heart disease, but anything, even gum disease, is associated with a higher risk.

Depression

Having depression or depressive symptoms significantly increases the risk of heart and related diseases, and also increases the risk of complications and death in people who already have heart disease. Depression is associated with a 1½ times higher rate of dying from coronary heart disease. Stress, loneliness, and lack of social support all contribute to depression, and are also associated with an increased risk of heart disease. It is important to note that good stress management, healthy diet, regular physical activity, and quality sleep are part of the treatment plan for depression, and we regularly "prescribe" these as self-care for our patients. However, these may not be enough. It's important for people to seek help from a healthcare provider, because they may also benefit from therapy and/or medications.

Sleep Disorders

Not enough sleep or low-quality sleep is clearly linked to many health problems, including heart disease. While not enough sleep is usually a life-style issue, low-quality sleep can be caused by obstructive sleep apnea (OSA), which is defined by frequent and long pauses in a person's breathing while he sleeps. He may notice that he wakes up gasping for air during the night and feels unusually tired and foggy in the day. Anyone watching him may hear snoring and become alarmed at the pauses in breathing and gasps for air. OSA is associated with high blood pressure, coronary heart disease, heart failure, arrhythmias, and strokes. Treating it with a machine (like a continuous positive airway pressure machine, or CPAP) not only cures sleepiness and clears brain fog, but it also helps lower blood pressure and improves heart function. OSA is often a result of obesity, and weight loss can reverse this condition.

Dietary Factors

The food we eat is an important risk factor that we can definitely control.

Processed Foods

The evidence is overwhelming, and the verdict is in: processed foods (flours and sugars in breads, pastas, cereals, snacks, basically anything in a box) are bad for us. Flours made from refined grains (like white flour) and sugars in breads, pastas, cereals, and many packaged snacks make our blood sugar spike, which triggers a surge of insulin, which then stores all that blood sugar as fat. Regularly eating these foods can lead to obesity, high blood pressure, high cholesterol, and diabetes. Not only that, but these foods get converted into toxic molecules that can directly damage the lining of our arteries. A diet high in refined grains and sugars is well associated with a significantly increased risk of premature death.

Sodium and Salt

Your body normally needs a small amount of sodium in order to function, about 500 mg daily. However, many people ingest over 3,400 mg a day, which can cause high blood pressure. The American Heart Association recommends no more than 2,300 mg daily (about the amount in a teaspoon of table salt), and less than 1,500 mg for some people. As most sodium is found in canned, processed, and fast foods, just eliminating these can reduce your sodium intake and your blood pressure significantly.

Meats

Mountains of evidence link eating meats to heart disease, cancer, and premature death, though some meats are riskier than others. Regularly eating cured, smoked, and processed meat products is particularly high-risk. Eating red meat is also associated with a higher risk of developing type 2 diabetes. This is thought to be an effect of heme iron (which is only found in animal meats).

We don't necessarily have to all go vegan, however. The traditional Mediterranean diet includes a lot of seafood, as well as some dairy, eggs, and chicken. (Regularly eating fish, particularly cold-water fatty fish like salmon, mackerel, sardines, and herring, is associated with a lower risk of heart disease.) As long as fruits, vegetables, beans and legumes, whole grains, and nuts and seeds are the main event, we can enjoy some meat.

Fats

The fat that clogs up our arteries is not necessarily from the fat that we eat. But some fats, especially trans fats, are clearly harmful for our bodies. These have been largely outlawed, though they are still sometimes found in small quantities. Even foods that are labeled "zero trans fats" may have a little—and even a little is bad—so be on the lookout for the words "hydrogenated" or "partially hydrogenated" on food labels.

Saturated fats are also solidly associated with a higher risk of heart disease. These are commonly found in fatty meats (bacon, sausage, deli meats, red meats); high-fat dairy (butter, cream); and baked goods. Though the messages in the press have been confusing, there is really no doubt about the risk. Avoiding these fats is key for heart health as long as they are replaced by healthy unsaturated fats, like those in nuts, seeds, avocados, fatty fish, and healthier oils (extra-virgin olive, safflower, canola, flaxseed, walnut, sesame). You'll learn more about all of this in Chapter 5.

Lifestyle Factors

Lifestyle refers to the way we live, and the daily choices we make can increase or decrease our risk for heart disease.

Smoking

Smoking is slam-dunk bad for your heart and circulatory system in many ways. Toxins in tobacco smoke cause increased blood pressure and stress on the heart. Toxin buildup damages cells, including the cells of our arteries, which promotes atherosclerosis (plaque buildup). Smoking is the number one biggest risk factor for heart disease, and the toxic effects cannot be counteracted by a healthy diet and active lifestyle. There is no evidence to suggest that vaping is any safer than smoking either. Not smoking is always a healthy lifestyle choice.

Sleep Deprivation

While sleep apnea and other sleep disorders can lead to sleep deprivation, so can our lifestyle. Insufficient sleep is directly linked to weight gain and obesity, high blood pressure, type 2 diabetes, heart disease, and premature death. These are likely all related: sleep deprivation causes increased inflammation and an exaggerated stress response (the fight-or-flight cascade of harmful hormones, like cortisol). Getting better sleep is an important lifestyle change goal.

How Much Sleep Do You Need?

Sleep researchers have published evidence-based recommendations for hours of sleep per day:

- Newborns: 14–17 hours
- Infants: 12–15 hours
- Toddlers: 11–14 hours
- Preschoolers: 10–13 hours
- School-aged children: 9–11 hours
- Adults: 7–9 hours
- Adults over age 65: 7–8 hours

*From the National Sleep Foundation's 2015 sleep duration recommendations

Inactivity

It is very well established that the more inactive a person is, the higher his risk of death, from just about any cause. Being inactive is the fourth leading cause of death in the world, after smoking, diabetes, and high blood pressure. Sitting is the new smoking: any prolonged periods of time spent sitting allow toxins to "sit" as well, damaging the blood vessels. Without regular exercise, blood vessels become stiff and more prone to sheer damage. Humans were meant to be moving, a lot, throughout the day. The good thing is, even a small amount of movement lowers risk for heart disease. Anything is better than nothing, and it all counts.

Stress

Stress (and all of the negative emotions that accompany stress) is one of the most important risk factors to understand and address—maybe the most important. If we don't manage stress well, we feel strong negative emotions, such as sadness, fear, and anger, which can progress to depression, anxiety, and hostility. These are all strongly associated with a high risk of heart disease. Loneliness and isolation exacerbate stress and contribute to illness and premature death.

Emotional stress triggers our body to release many hormones, including adrenaline and cortisol (the fight-or-flight response). Over time, this leads to high blood pressure, high blood sugars, inflammation, and toxic reactions, which in turn stress/strain and damage the heart and blood vessels. Unmanaged stress is associated with unhealthy coping behaviors, such as eating high-carbohydrate or sugary foods, overeating in general, binge-watching TV, playing video games, browsing the Internet, smoking, drinking, drugs… All of these can contribute to weight gain, high cholesterol, high blood pressure, and high blood sugars, and they further increase the risk of heart disease. There are many positive and healthy ways to cope with stress, which we will review in Chapter 3.

In summary, there are well-known risk factors for heart and related diseases. Though you can't change your genes, race, ethnicity, or gender, you can still lower your risk for heart disease through making healthy diet and lifestyle changes, and we'll learn how in Chapters 2 and 3.

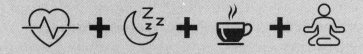

Chapter 2

Your Heart Is in Your Hands

IN THIS CHAPTER you'll see the proof that you can lower your risk of obesity, high blood pressure, high cholesterol, diabetes, heart disease, and even death through healthy diet and lifestyle changes, and the best way to do that is by targeting your everyday habits. You'll learn how stress management and behavioral strategies are key for making changes stick. Then you'll get an overview of the most important healthy habits.

Healthy Habits Help People Live Longer... Way Longer

What if there was a pill you could take to prolong your life by more than ten years? Research shows that adopting healthy lifestyle habits can do exactly this and without bad side effects.

Harvard researchers wanted to know what impact these diet and lifestyle habits had on life expectancy:

1. Eating a healthy diet (eating more fruits, vegetables, nuts, whole grains, and healthy fats; and eating less red and processed meats, sugary beverages, and high-salt and fatty foods)
2. Being regularly physically active (at least 30 minutes a day of moderate to vigorous activity)
3. Maintaining a healthy body weight (a normal body mass index [BMI])
4. Not ever smoking
5. Having moderate alcohol intake (no more than one drink daily, meaning 12 ounces of beer, 5 ounces of wine, or 1½ ounces of distilled spirits)

They looked at data from more than one hundred and twenty thousand people who had been studied for three to four decades, including self-reported habits, body measurements, and health outcomes. What they found was pretty remarkable: those who had all five diet and lifestyle habits lived significantly longer, on the order of fourteen years for women and twelve years for men! That's more than a decade of extra life without any pills or supplements. The more of these habits that people had, the longer they lived; having even just one habit prolonged life expectancy by two years. Adults who had none of these habits were far more likely to die young, mostly from cardiovascular disease or cancer.

As amazing as the findings of this study were, they basically confirmed the findings from other similar large observational studies: a few healthy habits can extend our lives significantly.

Longevity Lifestyle Lessons

There are certain places around the world where people tend to be healthier and live longer, to one hundred years or older. *National Geographic* reporter Dan Buettner organized a team of scientists and set out to study these healthy centenarians. His book, *The Blue Zones*, combines this series of interviews with the science of aging, with these lifestyle conclusions:

- Be active throughout the day, every day.
- Eat mostly plants, including fruits and vegetables, whole grains, legumes, and nuts.
- Eat mindfully, never overeating.
- Manage stress well.
- If you drink, limit drinking to just a bit of alcohol a day.
- Find a purpose for your own life.
- Make family a priority.
- Live within a community that supports you and these values.

While not a formal research study, the project conclusions are supported by science.

Diet and Lifestyle Changes Can Prevent Diabetes

Asking people what they eat, drink, and do and then relating it back to their health outcomes is one way to study the impact of diet and lifestyle. Another more scientifically rigorous approach is to take a bunch of people with risk factors for certain diseases, give some of them a diet and lifestyle change intervention, and see what happens. This is the strongest type of research study. One study like this was the Diabetes Prevention Program, which took people at risk for type 2 diabetes and gave them either a twenty-four-week diet and lifestyle intervention, a medication (metformin), or a placebo (a fake pill), to see if anything could lower their risk for developing diabetes.

The very comprehensive diet and lifestyle intervention had the goal of changing participants' daily habits and included: sixteen classes teaching basic nutrition and behavioral strategies for weight loss and physical activity, lifestyle coaches with frequent contact with participants, supervised physical activity sessions, and good clinical support for reinforcing an individualized plan. The reasoning behind this intervention was: we know that an unhealthy diet and lifestyle can cause type 2 diabetes, but can a healthy diet and lifestyle prevent it? Since type 2 diabetes is a huge risk factor for heart and related diseases, it's important to know if it can be avoided.

Perhaps not surprisingly the diet and lifestyle intervention was incredibly effective. After three years, the diet and lifestyle group had a 58 percent lower risk of developing diabetes than the placebo group. Participants aged sixty and older had an even better response, with a whopping 71 percent lower risk of developing diabetes. The diet and lifestyle effect lasted: even after ten years, those folks had a 34 percent lower risk of developing diabetes compared to the placebo group. Men, women, and all racial and ethnic groups had similar results (and almost half of participants represented racial and ethnic minorities). These results are not surprising to me nor to other doctors because we have all seen patients with prediabetes get their sugars down with diet, exercise, and weight loss alone.

Meanwhile, the medication group had a 31 percent lower risk of diabetes after three years and an 18 percent lower risk after ten years, which is also significant. It's perfectly all right to use medications along with diet and lifestyle changes, because each boosts the effect of the other. Studies looking at the combination of medication (metformin) with diet and lifestyle changes have shown powerful results.

Diabetes Prevention Programs Curriculum

Diet and lifestyle changes are so effective for diabetes prevention that as of April 2018, insurance companies are covering these programs for people at risk. The Centers for Disease Control and Prevention (CDC) has published the entire twenty-four-week curriculum on its website, and clinics around the country are establishing programs (check out www.cdc.gov/diabetes/prevention/index.html). Here is a summary:

During the first half of the program, you will learn to:

- Eat healthy without giving up all the foods you love
- Add physical activity to your life, even if you don't think you have time
- Deal with stress
- Cope with challenges that can derail your hard work—like how to choose healthy food when eating out
- Get back on track if you stray from your plan—because everyone slips now and then

In the second half of the program, you will enhance the skills you've learned so you can maintain the changes you've made. These sessions will review key ideas such as:

- Tracking your food and physical activity
- Setting goals
- Staying motivated
- Overcoming barriers

Take special note of the behavioral components. These aspects are critical to any successful diet and lifestyle change program, including one you create for yourself.

Diet and Lifestyle Changes Can Cure Diabetes

People can even reverse diabetes by changing their diet and lifestyle habits. In a study of more than three hundred participants who had already been diagnosed with type 2 diabetes, 46 percent of those who completed a twelve-month intensive diet and weight loss intervention—no medications, only nutrition and behavioral support—successfully reversed their diabetes, compared to 4 percent of those in the control group. As amazing as those results are, I have seen even more dramatic results in practice.

When my patient Preeti was diagnosed with type 2 diabetes, it was very advanced, with a hemoglobin A1c (HbA1c, the most common screening test for diabetes) of 11. That corresponds to an average blood sugar of 275. (For context, a normal average blood sugar should be under 126.) We were shocked: she had some risk factors for diabetes (ethnicity, overweight, and some family history) but no symptoms. Tests confirmed the diagnosis, and we had no choice but to start insulin injections along with metformin. I had little hope we would be able to discontinue either of these.

But Preeti was determined to make lifestyle changes. As she explained to me, "Prevention is more important than being treated with medicine, so there is a natural motivation not to be on medication if I can possibly avoid it." She followed a nutritionist's advice to avoid sugar and white flour, and eat more fruits and vegetables, lean proteins, beans, legumes, and whole grains. She also cut down on portion sizes, exercised every day for at least 30 minutes, and lost weight (20 pounds, from a BMI of 28 down to a BMI of 25).

All of that effort paid off: at a six-month follow-up appointment, her HbA1c was 5.8 (which corresponds to an average blood sugar of 120), and we were able to discontinue insulin altogether.

Preeti successfully treated her diabetes, but it didn't happen overnight. In her own words, "It takes time to make adjustments, and it's so important to have patience and be kind to yourself when you slip up." Like other patients who have made big lifestyle changes, it was not with diet and exercise alone, but also with trial and error, persistence, and trust in the process.

Behavioral Strategies for Beating Diabetes

Yes, learning about nutrition and physical activity is important. We're also seeing how critical behavioral strategies are for any successful diet and lifestyle change program. Things like dealing with stress, coping with challenges, getting back on track, staying motivated, and overcoming barriers, along with trial and error, having patience, and trust in the process can be essential for your success.

Diet and Lifestyle Change Can Cure Metabolic Syndrome

Metabolic syndrome is a cluster of problems (abdominal obesity, high blood pressure, abnormal cholesterol, and high blood sugars) very strongly associated with heart and related diseases. Cardiologist, researcher, and author Malissa Wood, MD, developed and studied a two-year comprehensive lifestyle change program for high-risk women in a socioeconomically disadvantaged city near Boston. The women had significant risk factors for heart disease—not only traditional risk factors like metabolic syndrome, but also high rates of stress, anxiety, and depression. The Health Awareness and Primary Prevention in Your Neighborhood (HAPPY) Heart Program incorporated nutrition; exercise; stress reduction classes (tai chi, yoga, and meditation); health coaching; and smoking cessation counseling. She found that among participants, the rate of metabolic syndrome fell from 65 percent to 35 percent at year one, and then to 28 percent at year two. Not only that, but their reported levels of stress, anxiety, and depression also significantly decreased.

The program was small (sixty-four women) but powerful. Many of the participants were financially challenged single mothers or grandmothers caring for kids, and they had a lot of stressors. In her published research, Wood cites the community support the program provided as perhaps one of its most important features: "In addition to becoming a place where the women came for education and exercise, the HAPPY Heart events and classes provided a psychologically therapeutic experience." In an interview, Wood emphasized the importance of good stress management as a foundation for successful behavioral change: "A lot of cardiologists go right to the LDL, the labs, the meds. Me? I ask, 'What's going on in your life right now?' Because no one is going to hear anything you have to say about nutrition and activity if you don't manage their stress first." Dr. Wood emphasizes that effective comprehensive lifestyle change programs should feature a strong behavioral component that helps participants to better manage stress. You're going to learn why this is so important in Chapter 3. If you're curious about the HAPPY Heart Program curriculum, much of it was published in Dr. Wood's book *Smart at Heart: A Holistic 10-Step Approach to Preventing and Healing Heart Disease for Women.*

Diet and Lifestyle Change Works

Lifestyle change programs can even be effective for people who already have heart disease. It was many decades ago that physician pioneer Dean Ornish, MD, first published research showing the positive impact a comprehensive lifestyle change program could have for patients with coronary heart disease. The initial amazing finding was that participants were able to make changes and sustain those changes over time. One of his early studies showed that after a year, program participants had a 37 percent lower LDL (the "bad" cholesterol) without taking cholesterol medications, far fewer episodes of chest pain (91 percent fewer), and measurable decreases in the blockages of their coronary heart disease, as compared to patients not in the program who had far more episodes of chest pain (165 percent more) and worsening of their coronary heart disease. The trial was so successful that it was extended another four years, and participants had even more improvements. The program has been replicated at other sites and has shown to be associated with many significant positive health outcomes, including improvements in BMI, cholesterol, blood pressure, HbA1c, exercise, and functional capacity, as well as less depression and hostility.

Dr. Ornish describes the program in his own words: "This lifestyle medicine program includes a whole-foods, plant-based diet (naturally low in fat and refined carbohydrates); stress management techniques (including yoga and meditation); moderate exercise (such as walking); and social support and community (love and intimacy). In short, eat well, move more, stress less, love more… Although the program is only nine weeks long, 85–90 percent of people are still following it after a year."

The irony that it is a natural, holistic, commonsense approach that works best now in this modern age is not lost on Ornish. "During the past forty years, we've used high-tech, state-of-the-art scientific measures to prove the power of these low-tech and low-cost interventions." Again, it's important to note that this successful program is about far more than diet and physical activity. The stress management and social support components are just as important. (Dr. Ornish has written extensively on this topic, and I highly recommend *The Spectrum*.)

Similar programs have been initiated by other groups, which also found positive health outcomes. Program costs can be high (between $3,800 and $4,441 by one 2012 study), but cost-benefit analyses show that participants have significantly fewer hospitalizations and lower overall healthcare costs.

While formal, comprehensive lifestyle change programs work well, they can be hard to find, require multiple in-person visits over a prolonged period (two months to two years), and are very expensive if insurance doesn't cover the costs. What is it about these programs that makes them work, and can we create our own program?

For Lasting Lifestyle Change, Change Habits

Lasting lifestyle change really means changing our everyday habits, well, for life. That's all it is. Sounds so simple, right? Let's try to better understand how habit change works.

We are only recently seeing high-quality health research studies targeting habits, but what we are seeing is safe, cheap, and effective. One recent study compared two weight loss programs: a psychological program that emphasized body image acceptance and a healthy relationship with food versus a habit-based program that helped participants break unhealthy habits while developing and maintaining healthy habits. Forty-three overweight or obese participants completed the twelve weeks of classes and group meetings. Surprisingly, both groups lost the same amount of weight—15 pounds. But the kicker was at follow-up. After six months, the psychological program participants gained 7 pounds (for a net loss of 8 pounds), while the habit-based participants lost 4 pounds (for a net loss of 19 pounds).

Another study of five hundred and twenty obese adults looked at a simple habit-based weight loss tool: a leaflet describing ten evidence-based health habits (called the "Ten Top Tips"), handed to patients and reviewed with a nurse at a single regular appointment. Half of the participants got the leaflet and a little logbook for self-monitoring, and the other half had a variety of other usual options, including referrals to weight loss centers and subscriptions to meal plans. The "Ten Top Tips" group lost an average of 5 pounds, and the weight loss was maintained after two years, without any further intervention.

Using a habit-based intervention for health is extremely promising, not only because such an approach has been shown to result in weight loss that was maintained over time, but also because it's inexpensive and doesn't involve medications or surgeries (so virtually no side effects or risks).

What Were Those Ten Habits, Anyway?

You're probably wondering what the "Ten Top Tips" habits for weight loss were. The original research and pamphlet are available for free online (see references at the end of the book), and I've included similar habits in the second part of the book. But here's a summary:

- Keep to your meal routine
- Go reduced fat
- Walk off the weight
- Pack a healthy snack
- Learn the labels
- Caution with your portions
- Up on your feet
- Think about your drinks
- Focus on your food
- Don't forget your five a day (five servings of fruits and vegetables a day minimum)

Medicine Takes a Lesson from Economics

Experts in economics and business already understand how important habits are and how powerful they can be—for profits. Marketers design their advertisements with the goal of making your choice of their product automatic. That's what brand loyalty is, after all: habit.

Business consultant Stephen Covey's classic book, *The 7 Habits of Highly Successful People: Powerful Lessons in Personal Change*, is largely based on his observations of and experience from working with organizations.

Investigative reporter Charles Duhigg's book *The Power of Habit: Why We Do What We Do in Life and Business* earned rave reviews from *The Wall Street Journal* and the *Financial Times*, and then enjoyed more than sixty weeks on *The New York Times* bestseller list. It was intended for business executives, but interestingly, the author also presents examples of how health habits can be changed for the better. In a follow-up interview, he described how researching and writing the book led him to change his own eating and exercising habits, and he lost 35 pounds.

Economists Christopher Payne and Rob Barnett applied the economic principles of "meta-rules and micro-habits" for their own lasting weight loss—more than 100 pounds combined. Their book, *The Economists' Diet: The Surprising Formula for Losing Weight and Keeping It Off*, has been hailed as a sensible, real-life plan. We in medicine, on the other hand, have been a little slow to recognize the power and potential of habits.

How Do Lifestyle Change Programs Change Habits?

The overarching goal of a successful lifestyle change program is to change the participant's daily habits, for good. We've seen that effective programs feature a strong behavioral component, which can include classes, health coaches, therapists, and group meetings; nutrition education with guidance from a dietitian; and a physical activity piece that often includes supervised exercise sessions or other activity monitoring. Here is a detailed overview of each of these components:

Behavioral Strategies

Changing habits isn't easy. This is why behavioral strategies are so critical. Successful lifestyle change programs emphasize the following behavioral areas:

Stress Management

Many stress-reducing techniques are associated with reductions in heart disease risk, especially exercise, mindfulness, meditation, and yoga. People who more effectively manage stress tend to have lower blood pressure, as well as lower rates of depression and anxiety. Most importantly, effective stress management is a key foundational skill for making healthy lifestyle changes stick. We're going to go into this in depth in Chapters 3 and 4.

Quality Sleep

Sleep problems, especially sleep apnea, are associated with a higher risk of heart disease, while treating sleep apnea lowers risk. Chronic sleep deprivation makes everything worse and causes weight gain. Getting enough sleep helps us better manage stress, as well as lose weight.

Social Support

People who have a solid support system have fewer health problems, perhaps because healthy relationships help us manage stress and avoid depression. This, in turn, can be protective against heart disease. There are other ways that family and friends can help us stay healthy. Studies show that eating meals with others helps us eat healthier and more slowly. Cultures that emphasize a leisurely sit-down family meal tend to have fewer chronic diseases overall. In addition, embarking on a lifestyle change plan with someone else helps us stick to the plan. Successful lifestyle change programs require classes and group meetings; some also feature family-style meals. The social support provided through these programs has been cited as one of the main reasons for their success.

Nutrition

Successful lifestyle change programs promote a healthy eating pattern, encouraging wholesome, natural, unprocessed foods, especially plants, and discouraging sugary, refined, or processed foods.

Plant-Based Diet

Hundreds of studies over decades prove that a plant-based diet is the healthiest diet. This means mostly fruits and vegetables; whole grains; legumes (beans, lentils, peas); and nuts and seeds. Studies show that eating ten servings of fruits and vegetables daily is associated with a 24 percent reduced risk of heart disease and 33 percent reduced risk of stroke. Even eating just two and a half servings daily can reduce the risk of developing heart disease by 16 percent, and of stroke specifically by 18 percent. That's half a grapefruit, an apple, and 3 tablespoons of peas. The fiber in fruits and vegetables binds cholesterol and fills us up, helping us eat fewer calories. Plus, fruits and veggies contain plant nutrients called *antioxidants*, which prevent and heal damage to blood vessels.

Most traditional diets (such as the Mediterranean diet) are associated with extremely low rates of heart and related diseases. The reason? Almost across the board, traditional diets are made up of mostly plants. They do not feature added sugar, refined flour, processed factory-made foods, cured/smoked or red meats, or fried foods. Though books and articles often refer to the Mediterranean diet, you can call it anything you like, as long as it's mostly vegetables, fruits, legumes, whole grains, nuts, and seeds. Seafood can also be a big component, and we'll go more into this in Chapter 5. Meanwhile, I recommend Dr. T. Colin Campbell and Dr. Thomas Campbell's *The China Study* and Dr. Michael Greger's *How Not to Die* as excellent plant-based diet informational resources.

Moderate Alcohol Intake

It's true that drinking a little bit every day significantly lowers the risk of heart disease. But there are a few potential problems: one, not everyone can safely drink alcohol. Two, drinking even a bit more than is recommended is bad for you and can cause a number of other health problems. Three, alcohol has calories and can make it harder for people to lose weight. Four, alcohol lowers inhibitions, which can lead to eating more. We're going to cover the pros and cons of alcohol more extensively in Chapter 5.

Healthy Weight

Having a healthy weight (BMI of 18–24) is associated with lower blood pressure, blood sugars, and cholesterol, as well as lower risks for heart disease. Weight loss through diet and lifestyle change is infinitely preferred over medications or surgeries, given their risks and costs. Most people who change their daily habits will lose weight. We'll cover this in Chapter 6.

Regular Physical Activity

Exercise of the body is exercise of the heart and blood vessels, too, making them flexible and stretchy, which keeps blood pressure down. Good blood flow brings in oxygen and healing molecules like antioxidants as it flushes out toxins. Exercise directly burns calories as well as builds muscle tone, which also boosts metabolism, helping us lose weight, prevent weight regain, and maintain a healthy weight. Even if there is no weight loss, exercise lowers blood sugars. The recommended goal is about 150 minutes of moderate physical activity per week, and we'll learn how to reach this goal in Chapter 7.

Not Smoking

This one goes without saying, but it really is important. Quitting smoking—at any age—decreases the risk of heart disease and increases life span. We'll cover how to quit smoking in Chapter 8.

Who's on Your Lifestyle Change Team?

Comprehensive lifestyle change programs involve a team of professionals. Even if you're not in a program, you may have access to many of these experts, depending on your medical history, insurance, and location. They may be able to provide resources and support for you.

Nutrition Experts

Many people can call themselves nutritionists, so it's important to understand that this can refer to a wide range of education, training, and clinical experience. For example, a nutritional consultant may have a high school degree and have passed an open-book certification exam, while a registered dietitian nutritionist (RDN) has a bachelor's degree, 1,000 or more hours of clinical training, and passed a national certification exam.

I spoke with Linda Delahanty, chief dietitian at the Massachusetts General Hospital Diabetes Center, who clarified the role of the nutrition expert: "It's the combination of knowledge of the evidence base— nutrition science, food composition—and counseling skills that make the best dietitian. In other words, someone who can skillfully combine the science and the art." She explains that "a registered dietitian provides an individual assessment of medical profile, lifestyle, current eating habits, and learning style, in order to create a personalized plan that focuses on the patient's nutrition priorities" and that developing the right plan is "a process that takes time....Dietitians typically spend an hour for the first session to do a thorough assessment, then schedule follow-up visits to educate, advise, and use behavioral counseling strategies to help people integrate these lifestyle changes into daily routines."

Mental Health Providers

Successful lifestyle change programs feature a strong behavioral component, usually involving mental health providers. There are many types, with widely varying education and training. Here are some common titles and what they mean:

- Health coach certification is available to almost anyone who takes a course, either in person or online.
- Licensed mental health counselor (LMHC) is a certification available to individuals with a master's degree in counseling, psychology, addictions, or therapy who have had clinical training and who have passed an exam.
- Licensed clinical social workers (LICSW) must have a master's degree in social work, do clinical training, and pass an exam; they are licensed in each state and entitled to work independently.
- Psychologists have an advanced degree such as PhD, PsyD, or EdD, have completed an internship and post-doctoral training, and have passed a national exam.
- Psychiatrists are physicians who have completed medical school and a psychiatry residency, passed a national certification exam, and obtained a state license. Psychiatrists work with people using a variety of counseling approaches and can also prescribe medications or other therapies.

If you are looking for a mental health provider to work with you, Massachusetts General Hospital psychologist Kathleen Ulman, who has more than four decades of clinical experience in individual and group psychotherapy, offered this advice: "There are many providers who are excellent therapists….It all depends on how much postgraduate study, supervision, and experience they have had. The important thing to know is that you should choose someone who is licensed and with whom you feel comfortable. Research shows that the most important factor in the success of psychotherapy or counseling is the relationship between the therapist and the patient."

Doctors

Many people can carry the title of "Doctor." It's important to find someone whose education and training meets your expectations and whose philosophy fits with yours.

Medical Doctors and Doctors of Osteopathic Medicine

These doctors have similar training. Both complete four years of college, plus four years of medical school, a clinical internship and residency program, and then pass a national certification exam and obtain a state license, as well as ongoing maintenance of certification requirements. Traditional MDs practice evidence-based medicine, following clinical guidelines and standards based on published research. DOs also practice musculoskeletal manipulation and tend to have a more holistic, individualized approach.

An MD or a DO can pursue additional training in these specialties:

- Obesity medicine specialists treat obesity using behavior modification, diet and lifestyle education, medications, and surgery.
- Lifestyle medicine specialists treat diseases using behavior modification, diet and lifestyle education, and health coaching.

- Functional medicine specialists identify and treat the root causes of disease using practices generally not based on scientific evidence but very individualized to the patient's symptoms.

Naturopaths and Chiropractors

Naturopaths and chiropractors are also doctors, with different education, training, and experience.

- Naturopathic physicians may use nutritional and botanical medicine, naturopathic manipulative therapy, and homeopathy to encourage the patient's own self-healing process.
- Chiropractors focus on the diagnosis and treatment of neuromuscular disorders, using manual adjustment and/or manipulation of the spine to reduce pain and improve the functionality of patients.

Physical Health Professionals

It can be helpful to work with an expert in physical health, but some titles that sound similar are actually very different:

- Physiatrists are MDs or DOs who have completed a residency training program in physical medicine and rehabilitation, which emphasizes restoring function and quality of life to patients with musculoskeletal or neurological problems. They may subspecialize in sports, brain or spinal cord injury, neuromuscular, or pain medicine.
- Physical therapists have completed a bachelor's degree and a three-year accredited doctoral program, and have passed a licensing exam. Physical therapists evaluate patients and develop treatment

plans using techniques to promote the ability to move, reduce pain, and restore function.

- Personal trainers have a high school degree and have completed a personal trainer certification program. They can oversee an individual's fitness program in a fitness facility or private setting.

More Lifestyle Change Resources Available to You

This book is not the first to combine evidence-based lifestyle recommendations along with behavioral change advice. Earlier in this chapter I presented the successful lifestyle change programs of Dean Ornish, MD, and recommended his book *The Spectrum*, as well of cardiologist Malissa Wood, MD, and her book *Smart at Heart*. I'd also like to highlight the work of other well-established, respected experts.

Walter Willett, MD, DrPH, is a physician, professor, researcher, and author who has been described as "the world's most influential nutritionist." While he has written loads of excellent articles and books, the most relevant one is *Eat, Drink, and Be Healthy: The Harvard Medical School Guide to Healthy Eating*, now in its second edition. In it he explains nutrition research and recommendations in a straightforward manner, also presenting some basic behavioral tips for healthy eating.

David Katz, MD, MPH, is a world-renowned expert in nutrition, obesity, and disease prevention. His book *Disease Proof: Slash Your Risk of Heart Disease, Cancer, Diabetes, and More—by 80 Percent* includes solid research explained clearly, as well as "skillpower," a number of practical behavioral tips and tools for everything from buying and preparing food, to navigating restaurants and socializing, to fitting in fitness.

These books emphasize that decades of science support the same, relatively simple diet: well-balanced and rich in fruits and vegetables, beans and legumes, whole grains, nuts and seeds, and maybe seafood, dark chocolate, and a little alcohol. They include healthy recipes and a lot of sound advice. I do not receive any benefits from providing these recommendations; rather, I know that we're all on the same passion-driven mission, and if my book doesn't work for you, then maybe theirs will. Heart disease is a huge problem, and it can only help to spread the word on how to prevent and treat it.

Go for Lifestyle Change! But Don't Stop Your Meds

Many diseases need to be managed with medications. Suddenly stopping some medications can be incredibly dangerous and even life-threatening. Please do not stop any meds without discussing with your doctor.

Sometimes, diet and lifestyle changes *plus* medications are the best choice. This combination can be a very powerful way to lower heart disease and stroke risk. Pills are not evil. They can be lifesaving. Medications to lower blood pressure, blood sugars, and cholesterol can help people a great deal, as can a simple daily aspirin.

Needing pills is not a fail. Pills will be far more effective, however, when combined with a healthy diet and lifestyle. Please work with your doctor and feel free to share this book with them!

You Can Create Your Own Lifestyle Change Program

In this chapter you saw the research supporting healthy lifestyle changes to prevent heart disease. Formal, comprehensive, intensive lifestyle change programs work very well, in large part because of the built-in behavioral component.

I have several patients who have created their own successful lifestyle change programs. In one case, a middle-aged patient had fallen into an unhealthy pattern, with steadily increasing weight, blood pressure, cholesterol, and sugars. "I wanted to get healthy, but I couldn't seem to get anywhere with it," remembered Vivienne. Her diet was poor, and she didn't exercise. "On weekday mornings I'd head down to the coffee shop for a slice of breakfast pizza or an egg sandwich." Her husband was a good cook who made big Italian dinners featuring garlic bread and lasagna. "We would eat the leftovers all week long," she recalled. "It was just what we did, and it was all bad habits….But that all changed when we found out about my heart."

An X-ray done for totally different reasons uncovered a surprise finding of coronary artery atherosclerosis, i.e., heart disease. Tests showed a blockage in one of the coronary arteries. It was caught early enough that she could still do something about it without needing any procedures or surgeries. The cardiologist prescribed some medications but also strongly advised a healthier diet and more exercise, which have been shown to reverse heart disease.

Vivienne began making changes. "I started with little things, and I kept going," starting with her weekday breakfast habit: "Now, I have a nice big fruit bowl and yogurt for breakfast or fruit and cottage cheese." Her husband got on board, as well: "He still cooks Italian meals, but we'll have chicken marsala or turkey tips. He steams veggies, and we pick on those all week." No more cheesy pasta leftovers.

She figured out how to add activity to her day, considering that she doesn't go to a gym. "When I'm cleaning my house, I'll put disco music on and dance around. I love disco!" she said with a laugh.

It's been a year and a half, and Vivienne has maintained a weight loss of more than 20 pounds. She's only on any medications because we know she has heart disease: a low-dose statin and a baby aspirin are all she takes. But even better? "I feel great, and I like the way I look too!"

I asked her if she had any advice for readers. She thought for a moment and then offered: "You have to have a good enough reason to begin with. Then it's just all these little things every day, and they add up." She mused, "Now, I don't even think about it."

It's become habit.

In the next chapter we'll learn more about science of habit and review some basic psychology and stress management skills so that you can change your habits and make the changes stick.

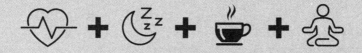

Chapter 3

How to Change Your Habits

IN CHAPTERS 1 AND 2, you learned what heart disease is, how it can be prevented (and even cured) by a healthy lifestyle, and that lasting lifestyle change can be achieved through targeting everyday habits. If you're thinking: "Okay, I know what to do and why, but now I need to know how!" then read on. In this chapter you'll learn about the science and psychology of habit, and how understanding our underlying psychology is critical for changing our habits. You'll see how stress, negative emotions, and thoughts can lead to bad habits and how positive coping skills can help change them, as well as a number of behavioral techniques to make those changes last.

What Is a Habit?

If you think that a habit is something that you do over and over so many times that it becomes automatic, then you're right. It's an action that we don't even think about, triggered by a cue in our environment. The decision-making part of our brain has very little to do with it. It's estimated that almost half of our daily actions are habits, everything from getting up out of bed, going to the bathroom, brushing our teeth, getting dressed, pouring our coffee, locking our door... When was the last time you had to go step-by-step in your mind, considering all the options and making decisions about every mundane action? What if every time you put your pants on, you had to think:

"Okay, first I unfold the pants, then grasp them at the waist, then step into the right pant leg, push my right leg through, put my right foot down, and then step into the left pant leg, push my left leg through, put my left foot down, then pull the pants up to the waist, button the top, zip the zipper..."

If everything you did involved step-by-step thinking, it would be hard to get anything done. You wouldn't be able to focus on other bigger things. This is why our brains evolved to form habits: so that we aren't constantly distracted by these step-by-step processes.

In his book *The Power of Habit*, Charles Duhigg uses a classic rat-in-a-maze model to illustrate how a basic habit is formed: A rat is placed at the beginning of a maze. It smells chocolate. It figures out the right path through the maze and then eats the chocolate. When the same rat is placed in the same maze again and again, it gets to the chocolate faster and faster. If it's given other lab-rat tasks for a few days or weeks and is then placed in the same maze, it will still go right for that chocolate. The rat now has a chocolate habit.

Humans have developed far more complex habit loops that involve way more steps. In my own experience, nothing highlights all those myriad complex steps like trying to teach them to a child.

Consider toilet training, for example. Some children grasp this hygienically necessary habit early on and without much coaching. Without embarrassing my kids too much, I'll just say that they did not exactly fall into that category. Yes, we wanted them to quickly realize that uncomfortable bladder and bowel sensations (the cue) meant run to the bathroom (the routine), so we bribed them with treats (reward). I'll spare you the details, but suffice it to say, there were a lot of tears and treats involved in establishing that habit loop. It was trial and error, which is typical for establishing any complex habit. As parents we struggled with what information and teaching needed to be combined with what coaching and reward in order to establish a new and consistent behavior. But just as the rat automatically remembers the way through the maze despite a hiatus, our kids (eventually) automatically remembered that when they feel the urge to go, they head to the bathroom. They don't need a reward from us anymore; the behavior has many of its own rewards, including physical (relief from the uncomfortable sensation) and social (society expects people not to soil themselves). As the habit loop is successfully repeated over and over, it becomes more and more established, and then, automatic.

Unfortunately, this is also true for bad habits.

Craving, Coping, and Habit

Most of us have firmly entrenched unhealthy habits that we would love to change.

"I need to have a bowl of ice cream after dinner," bemoaned Kevin, a patient of mine. "I crave ice cream. It makes me feel so good after a long stressful day at work. But if I could ditch that habit, I bet I'd lose ten pounds!"

In his book Duhigg points out that craving is a powerful driver of habits (particularly bad ones). When we're talking about lifestyle change, we need to understand that people crave things that help them cope with negative emotions. For Kevin, ice cream makes him feel good after a long stressful day at work. This is his habit: When he's feeling stress (cue), he gives in to his craving (routine), and it makes him feel good (reward). The problem is, his craving is not good for him.

Let's say Kevin decides to replace his unhealthy ice cream reward with a new healthy reward: naturally sweet, cold, fresh fruit. That should satisfy his craving, right? But he just can't seem to stop eating a bowl of ice cream after dinner. See, his very human habit loop is far more complex than the chocolate-eating rat's habit loop. Our negative emotions and unhealthy coping behaviors can seriously interfere with our ability to lose bad habits and form better habits. This is why most New Year's resolutions eventually fail and why lectures from our doctors, consults from dietitians, and sessions with our trainers don't work in the long term either. These things are not addressing the basic behavioral issues underlying our habits.

This is also why the formal intensive lifestyle change programs I described in Chapter 2 are so successful. They provide behavioral support, which can include therapy, health coaching, and group meetings. Unfortunately, those programs aren't a realistic option for most people since they can be hard to find, require a large time commitment, and can be expensive. But you don't necessarily need a formal program. You can, essentially, be your own health coach.

Coping Skills Are Critical for Lifestyle Change Success

Everyone experiences stressful situations. What's different from person to person is how they react and cope. Here's a situation you may relate to:

Imagine you're on the way to a meeting, but there's an unexpected delay, a horrible traffic jam. It's an important meeting, and you realize that you might miss it. As you sit in traffic, you may be feeling and thinking any of these negative things:

- Anger (frustration, irritation, blame, rage): "I can't believe I'm going to miss this important meeting because of this stupid unnecessary delay! This is outrageous! Someone needs to do something to fix this *now!*" [Bangs on steering wheel, beeps horn.]
- Fear (anxiety, worry, catastrophizing): "Oh my God. I might get in trouble for missing this meeting. I might get fired. I might not be able to find another job. Then I won't be able to pay my rent. I'll be homeless!"
- Sadness (helplessness, grief): "This always happens to me. It figures. I'm never going to get anywhere in life. Why bother trying. I'm a failure."
- Guilt (embarrassment, shame, self-criticism): "If I miss this meeting, I'm letting everyone down. What are people going to think? They're going to think I'm a slacker. If I had only left earlier…or I could have taken a different way. I'm such a stupid idiot."

How do you think you would react? Life is full of stressful events that may trigger negative emotions and thoughts, but how these impact you depends on how you cope.

Coping behaviors can be unhealthy or healthy. Unhealthy coping behaviors include eating or overeating unhealthy foods (like Kevin and his ice cream); bingeing on TV, Internet, or video games; overspending; smoking; drinking; gambling; and drugs. All these are behaviors that can lead to other problems (like addiction, which we will cover more in Chapter 8). People often develop very strong cravings for these behaviors.

Healthy coping behaviors include positive coping skills and can be learned. Even if you feel negative emotions about that traffic delay initially, these positive coping skills can turn them around:

- Putting it in perspective: "While this is not ideal, it's certainly not the end of the world. If this is the worst thing that happens to me today, then I'm a lucky person. There will be plenty more meetings, anyway."
- Understanding it's out of your control: "Well, there is nothing I can do about this delay. No sense in getting worked up about something when I can't do anything about it."
- Having a sense of humor: "I had just been thinking about how I'd love a little free time to catch up on other things! Funny how life works out."
- Putting a positive spin on it: "At least I don't have to sit in a stuffy conference room and listen to that boring presentation. I'd much rather have this quiet time to think. I've lucked out!"

There are other techniques that can help you in stressful moments:

- Deep breathing has been shown to bring down heart rate, blood pressure, and stress levels. Meditation is very similar to the

Relaxation response (discussed further in Chapter 4). There are meditation apps available that can be very helpful.

- Exercise, such as a brisk walk, is well-studied and can absolutely bring stress levels down in the moment, and for hours afterward. Regular exercise is an excellent stress management technique, always.

- Socializing and commiserating with others in the same predicament can alleviate negative emotions. Talking it out can be healthy, as long as it's not aggravating any negative emotions. The venting should lead to positive thoughts and not perpetuate negative ones.

We will learn how to incorporate these skills into your life in Chapter 4.

Protect Yourself from Stress

We just learned some positive coping skills for the moment that we're experiencing stress. We can also think ahead and prepare for future stressful times. This is especially important if you know that you have some unhealthy coping behaviors.

Stress eating as an unhealthy coping behavior is very common. In a 2013 survey of almost two thousand adults in the US, 38 percent reported overeating or eating unhealthy foods because they felt stress, and half reported doing so at least once a week. What can make this even more harmful is that people often crave sugary or carbohydrate-dense foods ("comfort foods") when they're stressed. Hormones such as cortisol, released during stress, cause more of that food to be stored as fat. This pattern of eating can lead to obesity, high blood pressure and cholesterol, diabetes, and heart disease. It's a big problem, but it can be solved.

Many people say: "It's hard to live healthy when you're feeling stressed." The opposite is also true: it's harder to feel stressed when you're living healthy. Getting good nutrition, exercise, and sleep, plus having a solid support system, are all critical components of a basic self-care regimen, which will help you when you're faced with life's challenges. We will learn ways we can incorporate self-care into our everyday life in Chapter 4.

Tips, Tricks, and Techniques for Making Habits Stick

Okay, we've emphasized stress management, and now we're moving on to practical techniques you can use for your lifestyle change efforts. Think about which ones may be helpful for you, and remember, trial and error is the norm.

Replace the Reward

In the case of my ice cream–eating patient, as soon as dinner is over, he craves ice cream. The reward is the sensation of sweet, which satisfies the craving. Maybe he can eat fresh fruit instead (once he's learned to better manage his stress). In this book we recommend aiming for ten servings of fruits and vegetables daily, so naturally sweet fresh fruit could be a win-win situation.

Rethink the Reward

Think about a bad habit that you want to go away. Why hasn't it vanished already? You've wanted it to, right? It hasn't gone because it's rewarding to you in some way. Think about the habit: what's it doing for you? In his book *The Power of Habit*, Charles Duhigg describes how he applied this technique to break a bad habit of heading to the office cafeteria most afternoons and eating a large cookie while chatting with colleagues. At first he thought the cookie was the reward. But he studied himself and realized it was actually the social interaction that he craved. Now he still heads to the cafeteria, but he buys a large tea and chats with his colleagues.

Now think about your bad habit. What is it really doing for you? Maybe you're really craving something else.

Make Rules

A habit is something that we do without thinking about it. By making rules for ourselves, we can help tap that automatic part of our brains. Rules have to be simple and straightforward, easy to follow. However, you can use more than one rule to help extinguish a bad habit.

I have a friend who lost 50 pounds through healthy diet and exercise. To do that she made up a bunch of rules. One was no snacking after dinner. To help her meet that goal, she "closed" the kitchen after eight p.m. and ended her food log for the day (by submitting the day's intake in an app). That was five years ago, but she still goes back to these rules when she feels like she's getting off track.

Change Your Identity

Nir Eyal, author and contributor at *Psychology Today*, describes how he became vegetarian: he declared himself one. He decided that eating meat was just something he didn't do. Incorporating his intent into this new identity made it a lot easier to resist eating meat. Saying, "I don't do that" is far more effective than saying, "That's something I'm trying not to do."

A patient of mine recently came in for her checkup and reported with delight that she had lost almost 10 pounds over a year by simply cutting out soda. "I just decided that I don't drink soda. I am a person who does not drink soda. It's poison for me." Making this a part of her identity helped her kick the habit.

Make a Bet You Don't Want to Lose

Behavioral scientists have long known that people are more likely to make a change if they have something to lose—rather than something to gain. In my office, this often takes the form of, "Okay, if your blood pressure is still abnormal in three months, we will have to start a medication at that point." Boy, is that motivating! Patients do not want to take medicine that they don't have to take (and I don't want to prescribe), and the risk of "losing" spurs them on.

Commitment Contract

Write down your goal in the form of a commitment contract. I do this with patients in the office sometimes, when we establish our goals for the next visit. There's something about writing something down that makes it "official." It also forces you to really think about and articulate what it is you'd like to accomplish. In order for this to work well, you should not be vague. "I will live healthy" is a big, admirable, yet vague goal. Break it down into smaller specific goals.

For example, for someone who is starting from scratch, I suggest that he doesn't write, "I will live healthy." Rather, divide that grand plan into different pieces, and then divide those up into specific actions:

"I commit to regular, daily physical activity. To do this:

- When I wake up, I will get out of bed and stretch before getting in the shower.
- When I am at work, I will set an alarm to remind me to stand up and walk around every 30 minutes.

- I will take a walk outside at lunch.
- When I am watching TV, I will stand up and move around at every commercial break."

And so on for each piece of the plan.

Tie a New Habit to an Existing One

It's so much easier to remember to do something if you're doing it at the same time as something you already always do. Follow me?

Let's say you want to meditate. You need to be sitting quietly to do this, so if you take the train, why not meditate while commuting to and from work? Or at your desk at work, as a midafternoon break? Or right before bedtime, after you brush your teeth? There are CDs, podcasts, and apps for this. (I use the Headspace app, which makes learning how to meditate very straightforward.) In these examples the meditation habit is tied to an existing part of your regular routine.

I have a patient who used to get bored while walking her dog. Then she discovered podcasts—uplifting or funny ones. Now she downloads positive podcasts and thoroughly enjoys her dog-walks. She's actually getting in three healthy habits at the same time: Walking, pet therapy, and feeling positive!

Repeat, Repeat, Repeat

Just repeating the same habit can help make it stick. Several years ago (and admittedly after being rescued from a broken elevator) I decided to always take the stairs. After all, stair-climbing is excellent exercise, and on workdays I may not have time to exercise otherwise.

It was hard at first. And kind of annoying. When I was with people who couldn't or wouldn't take the stairs, we had to figure out where to meet, and then they had to wait for me. But I stuck with it. It's now a running joke among my students and colleagues (though they are sometimes inspired to take the stairs with me, up to a certain number of floors). Me, I don't even think about it anymore.

How long does it take for a new behavior to become habit? Popular belief says twenty-one days, but it's different for everyone and can take way longer than that. Researchers trying to answer this very question found that it took anywhere between eighteen days to eight months, with the average being about eight weeks.

Bringing Habit Science Home

If you enjoyed these habit-forming tips, then you may enjoy some more reading on the topic. When writer/researcher Gretchen Rubin decided to live a healthier lifestyle, she studied the process and wrote a book: *Better Than Before: What I Learned about Making and Breaking Habits—To Sleep More, Quit Sugar, Procrastinate Less, and Generally Build a Happier Life.* There are several practical chapters: the one about Loophole-Spotting focuses on the unhelpful thought patterns that can derail our best-laid plans. There's the Tomorrow Loophole ("It doesn't matter what I eat now, because I'm starting a diet tomorrow"); the This Doesn't Count Loophole ("I'm on vacation" and "It's holiday season"); and the always slippery Moral Licensing Loophole ("I went running today, so I've earned a few beers"). Her suggestions are generally evidence-based, eminently doable, and the book is a fun read.

What's Next?

In Part 1, we've reviewed the basics of heart and habit science, and learned how to lay the foundation for change, how to anticipate common challenges, and which techniques will make habits stick.

In Part 2, you'll learn one hundred evidence-based healthy habits for your heart. You may be wondering what "evidence-based" means. Before a doctor can recommend anything to a patient, we need to have solid evidence that it's safe and effective. This is what separates a medical doctor from a witch doctor. Treatments need to be studied by researchers; then researchers have to publish what they did, how they did it, and what results they got. Keep in mind that even though the media loves to report on research that shows something new or unexpected, one study by itself is not enough to change guidelines or treatments. In addition, not all research is done well. We like to see lots of quality studies before coming to conclusions.

The one hundred habits listed in Part 2 are backed by solid research and will lower your risk of developing heart disease (and its cronies, like strokes and dementia). There are yummy recipes too. Let's go!

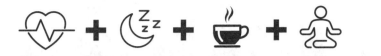

PART 2
Habits for Heart Health

- **Chapter 4: Change Your Life: Foundational Habits** will build up your positive coping skills using effective stress management techniques, as well as help you improve your sleep and strengthen your social support.
- **Chapter 5: Eat for Your Life: Nutrition Habits** will give a comprehensive, well-researched, and detailed review of the latest heart-healthy diet and eating information, ideas for how to incorporate this into your daily life, plus recipe suggestions.
- **Chapter 6: Lose Weight for Good: Healthy Weight Loss Habits** will provide safe, effective, and evidence-based weight loss advice; practical and doable ideas; and recipe suggestions.
- **Chapter 7: Run (Walk, Dance, Garden...) for Your Life: Activity Habits** will help you increase your activity level effectively and painlessly.
- **Chapter 8: Addressing Heart-Harmful Habits** will show how habit and addiction can overlap and includes sections on smoking, different types of overeating, and electronics overuse.

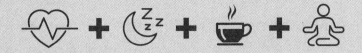

Chapter 4

Change Your Life: Foundational Habits

IF YOU'VE RECENTLY decided to change your life-style habits, then this chapter will provide the foundation for your success.

But if you've already been trying, you may be thinking, "I know what to do, I just need to do it." This is a frustration that a lot of people feel. They're trying, but it's not working. That may be because a diet and exercise plan is only part of the lifestyle change equation. If you've been feeling frustrated, then you may need a diet and exercise plan *plus* a behavior change plan. This chapter is full of specific behavioral actions, most of them very small and yet still very significant. You can pick and choose which ones work best for you, and hopefully, you'll get the boost that you need.

Stress Management Habits for Your Heart

We've learned how good stress management is critical for successful behavior change. Here are some practical stress management suggestions to put into action.

1. Create a Self-Care Schedule

If you want to make lasting healthy lifestyle changes, then you need to prioritize *you*. "We as a society do not take self-care seriously enough," says Stephanie Eisenstat, MD, senior physician at Massachusetts General Hospital and former director of the Diabetes Care Collaborative. She has more than a decade of experience running lifestyle change groups and describes: "People cry when I tell them that it's okay to take care of themselves. People break down into tears. There's so much emotion around that. For some people, their inner voice has been saying, 'I'm no good, I'm not worth it,' and we need to help them rewrite that script." In addition, many people put the well-being of others ahead of themselves. They may be healthcare providers, first responders, or maybe they're caring for kids or elderly relatives.

A huge part of any successful lifestyle change program is helping people understand that it's okay to take care of themselves. If you're a caregiver, your ability to take care of the people around you depends on your own health and well-being, so you need to be at the top of your to-do list.

Let's make that list. What are the things that make you feel good and that are also good for you? Maybe it's getting a little activity in most days (or even some days is fine). Or maybe it's going to yoga, or church, or volunteering, or getting a massage once a week. Don't just pencil it in; set it in stone. Make that time sacred.

Tips to Make the Habit Stick

- Pick one self-care activity every week that will be set in stone on your schedule. Enter it as a weekly recurring event on your calendar.

- Decide what you'll tell people if they ask what you're doing at that time. You can tell them you've got a doctor's appointment. If what you do during that time helps you be at your best, then it's even more important than a doctor's appointment!

- If there is someone who can accompany you on your self-care activity, ask her to join you and make it a plan. Maybe it's walking in the morning or at lunch or booking a therapeutic massage. Whatever it is, promising someone else that you'll be there can help you stick to your self-care routine.

- Start small. If you're not accustomed to taking time for yourself, it's best to begin with something very easy. Is there a beautiful view anywhere near you? A pond, waterfront…even a view of the city from an office window counts. Go there and take in the view, breathe deeply, and stretch a bit. This brief, relaxing minute is all yours.

- If you tend to abandon yourself and put others first, or you aren't convinced you are worth the effort, then you may benefit from talking to a mental health professional. The websites www.psychologytoday.com/ and www.psychcentral.com/ have solid mental health information and listings of credentialed therapists by city and state, and I usually suggest reaching out to a few to see who may be a better fit. There are even online, phone, and texting options, like www.talkspace.com/ and www.betterhelp.com/.

2. Listen to Music

Several studies have shown that people who listen to soothing music can experience significant physiological benefits, including lower stress levels and blood pressure. It needs to be calming music, though. In a 2015 Italian study, sixty participants with known coronary heart disease listened to Mozart, The Beatles, or the news. Those who listened to Mozart had a 7.2-point drop in their systolic blood pressure compared to the other groups. In a 2016 German study, sixty participants listened to Mozart, Strauss, or ABBA. People who listened to Mozart and Strauss had a 5-point drop in their systolic blood pressure, as well as slight drops in diastolic pressure and heart rate; all three groups had a significant drop in cortisol levels (a stress hormone).

Further reading on this suggests that if the music is soothing (and not stimulating) to you, it will have a beneficial effect on your body. Pick music that you find calming and that ideally does not have words. If it's relaxing music to your ears, regardless of whether it's Latin jazz, chill hip-hop, lounge electronica, or classical orchestral, it should be effective for stress reduction.

Tips to Make the Habit Stick

- Make it easy to listen to calming music when you need to. If you listen to music on your smartphone or computer, then when you have some time, pull together a stress-reduction playlist. Title it "relax" or something that you will recognize quickly. If you listen to CDs, have all of your relaxing ones close at hand.
- Where are you when you feel stressed? Maybe it's on your commute to work or at work. Maybe it's when you get home, and you see all the housework and chores that need to be done. These are good times to put on some relaxing music. This can lower your heart rate, blood pressure, and stress hormones when you need it most.

3. Breathe. Deeply. Seriously.

The deep breathing thing is really a thing. This has been studied, a lot. As a matter of fact, there are books about this technique, ranging from deep breathing to address specific conditions like stress to breathing for your general health and well-being. Herbert Benson, MD, conducted some of the original research on how simple deep breathing could lower heart rate, blood pressure, and stress levels. He developed an easy technique called *the Relaxation Response*, which was first described in his 1975 book by the same name, and has been widely disseminated in the years since. The Relaxation Response is very similar to meditation but perhaps more straightforward. For those who use it regularly, it is more effective than medications. Here is an abridged version:

- Sit quietly in a chair in a comfortable position and close your eyes.
- Relax your muscles, beginning at your feet and progressing up to your face.
- Breathe through your nose. As you breathe out, say a simple word silently to yourself, something like "calm" or "love" or "one." For example, breathe in, and then out, saying "one." Repeat.
- When distracting thoughts occur, as they will, don't worry about it. Just let them go and return to your breathing and saying your word on the exhale.
- Continue for anywhere between 1 and 20 minutes.
- When you finish, sit quietly, open your eyes, and go on with your day, feeling refreshed and relaxed.

The Relaxation Response technique has been studied for decades and is associated with lower stress levels and lower blood pressure. It gets easier with practice. Try to practice once a day, so that in a time of stress, when you really need it, you'll be able to relax easily.

Tips to Make the Habit Stick

- Find a good time when a few minutes of deep breathing (Relaxation Response or some other technique) may work well for you. This can be anywhere, anytime, really: sitting at your desk, on the train, before bed…even driving, though you'd want to keep your eyes open.
- Schedule breathing sessions in your calendar. Make it official. Make it something you just do. Set an alarm even. Bring your blood pressure down the natural way.
- Start with 1 minute, just 1 minute, of deep, mindful breathing. Increase over time, but if you don't have a lot of time, a minute is still fine.

4. Think Positive, Feel Positive

We've known for ages that poor stress management and negative emotions leading to depression and hostility are associated with a higher risk of heart disease. Here's the thing: the opposite is also proving to be the case. Positive emotions such as optimism and an overall sense of well-being are associated with a lower risk of heart disease and longer life, even in people who have heart disease. One 2011 English study of eight thousand people found that those with high levels of optimism and sense of well-being had a 30 percent lower risk of developing heart disease. Studies suggest that this may be due to positive emotions boosting our immune response and blunting the stress response. Other studies show that having positive emotions is protective against stress. Optimism and a sense of well-being are associated with lower stress hormones and inflammation, as well as lower heart rate and blood pressure.

Tips to Make the Habit Stick

- Get in the habit of "flipping" negative situations around. Stuck in traffic? Instead of fuming, look at it as a great opportunity to make a mental to-do list, listen to a podcast you've been saving, or check out a new album. The store didn't have what you need, and you walked all that way? Think of all the steps you got! You're that much closer to your exercise goal for the day.

- Having trouble seeing the bright side? Imagine how things could be worse. For many people, they are. Be thankful and grateful that your situation isn't as bad as it could be.

- Still can't think positive? You can still *feel* positive. Listen to a funny show or podcast, or even better, read a humorous book. Laugh. Laughing is well known to make people feel significantly more positive.

5. Fake It 'til You Make It

Even if you feel unhappy and stressed, and no amount of positive thinking is working, just pretending you're happy works. Research supports this. In one fun study, researchers divided one hundred and seventy participants into three groups and manipulated their faces into either a neutral expression, a smile involving only the corners of the mouth (a "fake" smile), or a smile involving the eyes as well (a "natural" smile). All the participants were then asked to complete stressful tasks, and their heart rates were measured. The groups whose faces were manipulated into smiles had lower heart rates than the group with a neutral expression. It's hypothesized that when your brain senses your face muscles smiling, it triggers brain pathways usually associated with real smiling, thus activating a "happy" hormone cascade. So even if you're feeling stressed and sad, smile. It will help you feel less stressed!

Tips to Make the Habit Stick

- When you find yourself frowning or scowling, force your face into a smile. Even if it's a mouth-only fake smile, it will help.
- When you're feeling tense, stretch your facial muscles into that smile shape. This is especially effective when you're working at a desk or driving, because that's when head and neck muscles can become very tense.

6. Exercise Is Anti-Stress Medicine

Exercise, any exercise, is a safe and effective stress management tool. In the American Psychological Association's 2013 Stress in America survey of almost two thousand adults, 30 percent said that exercise made them feel less stressed, 35 percent said exercise put them in a good mood, and 53 percent said they feel good about themselves after exercising. Not only that, but exercise benefits us in other ways, most of which involve our heart health. Exercise boosts our metabolism; increases muscle tone; and helps heal the arteries of the heart, brain, and body.

How much of what type of exercise is needed in order to see a stress reduction benefit? Multiple research studies over the years have shown that more physical activity makes people feel less stressed, and 30 minutes of brisk walking four or five days per week should be a minimum goal. Of course, that doesn't mean that's what you have to do, especially right off the bat. Any amount helps, and any activity counts.

Tips to Make the Habit Stick

- Think about what activities you enjoy. If you hate, loathe, and despise running, then, please, don't run. Make a mental list and refer to it often: "I like to do X, X, and X for fun." Every week (or day) think, "Have I done X yet? How can I fit some X in?"
- Schedule activity into your regular weekly routine. Active time is as important to your health and well-being as a medication or a doctor's appointment.
- Any bodily movement counts. Look for opportunities to move your body throughout your day: get up and talk to someone instead of texting or emailing; park farther away when you drive somewhere; pace while you're talking on the phone.

7. Volunteer

Plenty of observational research shows that volunteering is associated with improved emotional well-being, life satisfaction, and reduced depression. More recent research shows that volunteering is associated with lower stress hormone levels. In a study of three hundred and forty adults, cortisol levels were significantly lower on days they did volunteer work. The authors concluded, "Volunteer programs designed to help others in need may be considered as an intervention strategy for individuals living under stressful conditions." Volunteering your time for a charitable cause can be a win-win strategy: good for you, good for the cause.

A lot of people feel that they don't have the time to volunteer. However, many volunteer opportunities require a small time commitment on a weekly, monthly, or even sporadic basis. Some jobs can be done from home! Charities are often looking for people to help with their websites or provide other technical support.

Tips to Make the Habit Stick

- Think about the causes you'd like to support and reach out to a bunch. Try out a few. One may be a better fit for you and your schedule. I care for the cats at a local animal shelter every Thursday morning, and that time is essential for my own well-being. It's good for the cats, but it's even better for me!
- If you have a family, think about volunteer opportunities for all of you. Regularly volunteering is a powerful educational tool for kids. It teaches them so much, from the importance of an individual's efforts toward the greater good, to the reality of the world around them, to basic responsibilities... Volunteering with your kids can be a win-win-win: good for you, good for the cause, and good for

your kids. Food pantries, soup kitchens, and animal shelters commonly allow families to volunteer.

- No time? That's okay. Think of a cause you feel strongly about and offer virtual support. Hold an office or Facebook fundraiser (those can raise a lot of money!). Throwing a birthday party? Whether it's for you or for your kids, ask for donations to your favorite charity instead of gifts.

8. Keep a Journal...a Gratitude Journal, That Is

In one study, researchers divided healthy and chronically ill people into groups that each had different daily journaling assignments for several weeks. Those who were asked to write down a few things for which they were grateful had a significantly increased sense of well-being and improved mood by the end. Another study applied this same research framework to fifty adults with heart failure. After eight weeks, the daily gratitude journaling group had significantly lower levels of inflammation and heart response to stress, as well as a sense of gratitude. Making a daily habit of recognizing a few things for which you are grateful is an excellent healthy coping strategy and can have significant psychological and physical benefits.

Tips to Make the Habit Stick

- In the first study I mentioned, the official instructions were: "For the next eight weeks you will be asked to record 3–5 things for which you are grateful on a daily basis. Think back over your day and include anything, however small or great, that was a source of gratitude that day. Make the list personal, and try to think of different things each day." You can try this as well.
- If you have kids, have them do this daily exercise as well. Teaching kids gratitude is so important. This is a win-win!
- Don't have time to write it down? That's fine. In your head, any time of day, think of a few things for which you are grateful. That counts.

9. Grow a Garden

A 2016 analysis of twenty-two research studies found that gardening was associated with multiple significant psychological benefits, including lower risk of depression or anxiety and increases in life satisfaction, quality of life, and sense of community. (It also resulted in a lower BMI.) A variety of gardening situations from small urban patio gardens to large community plots were studied, and methods included comparing people before they gardened to afterward, or comparing gardeners to nongardeners. It turns out that gardening is good for our mental and physical health.

Tips to Make the Habit Stick

- You can order an inexpensive and easy-to-assemble raised garden kit or large planters online, as well as gardening soil and seeds (or even seedlings). Once you have the setup, it's just a matter of watering and weeding.
- No outdoor space? An indoor herb garden gives you the well-being of gardening and the bonus of fresh, inexpensive herbs for your cooking (and tea!).

10. Declutter Your Space

Your space refers to your home and work areas and your vehicle as well. Think about decluttering and reorganizing to make everything as clean and simple as possible. This has the amazing effect of helping you declutter and reorganize your entire life.

Tips to Make the Habit Stick

- Here is a strategy used by professional organizers: Pick one space and enter it with two garbage bags. One is for trash; one is for donating. Consider every item within the space, asking yourself these questions:
  - Is it useful? If you think it's useful, have you used it within the past year? If not it's probably not useful. If your reaction is, "But it might be someday" then it's probably clutter. Consider donating it so it can be useful to someone else.
  - Is it something precious to you, that brings you joy? Maybe it's a piece of art that you love to contemplate or a sculpture your kid made years ago. It's perfectly okay to save these precious items. But if it's something that you feel obligated to keep around, like a gift you don't care for, then it's clutter. Trash or donate.
  - Does it belong to someone else? Return borrowed items or ask people to come and get them.
- Many charity organizations will pick up items for donation. You can usually schedule a pickup time online and leave items on your front stoop. Bonus: donations to a charity organization are tax deductible!
- Organize just one small space, like a drawer. Or divide your closet into multiple smaller areas (like right side, left side, floor, overhead shelf) and tackle each area separately. Promise to keep at it daily. Your closet will be decluttered and reorganized within a week.

11. Learn to Say No

This is a short tip, but it's incredibly important for your self-care (and sanity). It can be hard to say "No" when people ask you to take on a project or responsibility. After all, they're telling you that they need your knowledge and expertise. But every time you're asked to do something, consider: is it something that you really want to do? Is it in line with your goals for you, your career, or your family? It's okay—and sometimes really necessary—to say no to requests that aren't in line with your goals. Taking on tasks, projects, and responsibilities that aren't good for you, your career, or your family is a harmful drain on your precious time and energy and an obstacle to your good health. Saying no is a critical self-care skill.

Tips to Make the Habit Stick

- Look at your schedule. Is there anything on there that annoys or irritates you, that you regret taking on, or that you dread? Let it go.
- When people ask you if you can take something on, it's okay to say NO. But if you don't feel confident enough to say no right away, just say you'll think about it, and then say no later.

12. Forgive

Anger, hostility, and vengefulness are really, really bad for you. There is scientific evidence that these negative emotions cause stress on the mind and body, and they are highly associated with an increased risk of heart disease and complications from heart disease. Reliving events, holding anger against the person, and ruminating on revenge cause more harm to you than to anyone else. It follows, of course, that being able to let go of these harmful emotions could be extremely beneficial, and studies show that it is. Forgiving the offender is not at all saying that the acts the person committed were acceptable. It is just letting go of the negative, damaging emotions. Forgiveness, including self-compassion and loving-kindness meditation, are common and important therapy approaches that are practiced widely, particularly for victims of childhood abuse, domestic violence, or people suffering from post-traumatic stress disorder (PTSD). For these situations, the forgiveness approach is best mediated by an experienced, licensed mental health professional.

Tips to Make the Habit Stick

- The next time someone annoys or irritates you, once the event is managed, let it go. Make a conscious effort not to relive it by talking about it or ruminating on it, because that brings all the negative emotions back again and again. For example, if someone says something mean or insulting, it's perfectly all right to let him know that his actions are not welcome. Once you've made your feelings known, let it go, and you will be a lot happier.
- If you have a hard time letting things go after an event, try writing about it. A useful technique is to write down everything you feel and that you wish you could say or do. Don't actually say or do any

of it. Write it down and then rip up/burn/shred that piece of paper. The negativity is now symbolically gone. Poof.

- Still harboring anger? Reliving old arguments? Thinking of good comebacks? All that negativity is really bad for your heart and soul. A mental health professional can help.
- For anyone who has been the victim of abuse, this forgiveness approach is complicated and should be guided by a very experienced, licensed mental health professional.

13. Cuddle a Kitten
(or Pet a Puppy or Hug a Bunny...)

The human-animal bond is well recognized by science. Animal-assisted therapy has been shown to reduce stress, anxiety, and loneliness; improve mood and general well-being; and enhance socialization. Pet owners can attest to this. But you can experience the "Pet Effect" even if you don't own your own animal companion. In addition to enjoying other people's pets, you could consider volunteering at an animal shelter (and thus getting in Habit #7 as well!). Even if your schedule is nuts, shelters often keep a list of volunteers to step in on occasion. One fun seasonal position is "kitten cuddler": people who come in and help socialize kittens so they become comfortable with humans before they get adopted. What could be more stress relieving than cuddling kittens—and knowing you're doing a good deed at the same time?

Tips to Make the Habit Stick

- If you own a pet, realize how good they are for your soul. Throw a ball for your dog, shine a laser-light for your cat, play hide-and-seek with your rabbit (I understand that's a thing).
- Do a quick online search to see what animal shelters are in your area and apply to be a volunteer. Check them out (most have a volunteer orientation) to see if they're good matches.

14. Walk in Nature

A substantial body of research shows that spending time in nature, or "green spaces," is associated with significantly lower stress levels. In one recent study, more than one hundred participants spent about an hour in one of three spaces: a natural park with forest and fields, an urban park with benches and paths, or an indoor recreation center with a running track and exercise equipment. The natural park group was the only group with reported reduced stress and increased joy, as well as reduced stress hormone levels. Scientists have several theories to explain this phenomenon: one is that being in nature allows our brains to relax. We're bombarded by technology and unnatural noises all day long. Being in nature may be a massive relief to our poor overstimulated neuronal pathways. Another is that being in nature triggers primitive relaxation pathways in our brain, based on how we evolved. Our ancestors needed to know when they could relax, and being in wide open spaces with access to water was relaxing because they could see that there were no predators and knew they would have water to drink. Maybe this is why we still feel a deep sense of satisfaction when we take in a beautiful view.

Tips to Make the Habit Stick

- If you are able to spend time during your regular workday in a natural setting, make that a priority. Maybe you can walk through a park on the way to or from work or sit and have lunch under a tree. Even if it's looking out an office window overlooking trees, grass, and maybe a body of water, that can provide benefit.
- If you have the option of being active in a natural setting, like walking in a forest, through a park, or along water, choose that option. It's a double benefit: activity and green space!

15. Get a Massage

Moderate-pressure massage has been associated with body and mind benefits ranging from reduced depression and anxiety, to lower heart rate and blood pressure, to decreased stress hormone levels. It can even alter brain wave patterns similar to the Relaxation Response. The National Center for Complementary and Integrative Health (a division of the US government's National Institutes of Health) lists conditions for which there is more solid evidence that massage is beneficial. These include chronic pain syndromes (neck and back pain) and depression, which are often stress-related. This is important because some insurance will cover treatments for these conditions. Massage treatments can be offered by massage therapists, as well as certain chiropractors and physical therapists. In the US, most states require massage therapists to meet standards of education, certification, and licensure. You can find a massage therapist near you through www.amtamassage.org/findamassage/index.html or www.abmp .com/public.

Tips to Make the Habit Stick

- Massage treatments should be regular and ongoing in order for you to derive consistent and ongoing benefits. If you find massage helpful for you and are able to book regular treatments, make it a priority in your schedule.
- Of course professional treatment with a licensed provider is ideal, but even a massage from a partner or self-massage can be beneficial. If you work at a computer or drive for hours, take regular breaks to stretch and press on any tight, sore muscles.

16. Have a Cup of Tea

Teas, which you'll learn more about in Chapter 5, are packed with polyphenols, antioxidant plant nutrients that help detoxify and heal your body. These amazing molecules counteract stress by blunting the body's cardiovascular response to stress hormones. They lower heart rate and blood pressure, as well as neutralize toxins, all of which help keep your arteries and heart healthy. While green and black teas are loaded with these plant nutrients, there are plenty of polyphenols in herbal teas as well. Some herbal teas popular for stress relief are worth trying, especially if you don't want any caffeine: mint, chamomile, and lemon.

Tips to Make the Habit Stick

- If you find that you benefit from particular teas, bring some with you to work or keep them with you while traveling. Hot water is easy to find, but the particular tea you like, not so much. This can also be quite economical, since one cup of tea at a restaurant or coffee shop will cost you at least $1 or $2, while a box of twenty tea bags can cost $3 or $4 total.
- Take tea breaks. If you work long hours at a desk, schedule a stretch, walk, and tea break. If your office doesn't have an electric teakettle, consider bringing one in, along with your favorite tea bags. This can be part of your effective yet economical daily stress-relief session.

17. Protect Yourself from Stressful People

Some people are so stressed that it spills over from their lives into yours. They may be constant complainers, always the victim in yet another drama. Maybe they're judgmental and critical of you and always make you feel bad about yourself. If you feel drained and down or angry and insulted after spending time with someone, then if at all possible, avoid that person. If not, then consider other proactive strategies. If it's a Negative Nellie dumping her latest woe on you, and you feel a reply is required, you can always nod and murmur, "Must be difficult; I'm so sorry," and then pretend you've got a meeting. Is this someone at work? Avoid direct contact as much as possible and communicate via impersonal (and always professional) emails. Is this an acquaintance or relative you have to see at holidays? If you must engage, keep it light: weather and sports or other benign, impersonal topics only. If he tries to engage you, which he likely will, ignore or dodge. A polite nonreaction followed by a quick change of subject works well and discourages future interaction. The key is to stay neutral and impassive. Toxic people thrive when they can spread their poison, and reacting to them or engaging with them is drinking their poison. Just say no.

Tips to Make the Habit Stick

- Is there anyone in your life who makes you feel drained, down, angry, or bad? Be proactive. Think of strategies and phrases you can use to avoid, dodge, distract, and discourage her. Have a plan.
- You do not need to provide any explanations or apologies, because you're being professional and polite. You're neutral like Switzerland. Do not engage.

- If these techniques don't work, create emotional distance. A psychiatrist colleague once pointed out that most of these negative, destructive people have their own significant issues, and we can use a combination of pity and patience to let their words roll off our backs. The way he explained it: "If a crazy person points at you and says, 'You're an eggplant,' how do you react? You'd probably feel sorry for them, shrug, and walk away. It's the same thing if someone points at you and says, 'You're dumb' or 'You're ugly.' It's their problem, not yours. Feel sorry for them and walk away." I'd like to point out that the psychiatrist used the word *crazy*, not me. But the point is a good one, and I use this technique also.

- Stressful people can be abusive people. It's important to note that abuse doesn't have to involve hitting or other physical violence. If there is someone in your life who puts you down or says hurtful things, tries to control you, or makes you feel afraid, that is abuse. If you think that you may be in an abusive relationship, please talk to someone about it. There are many resources, and in the United States, we have the National Domestic Violence Hotline. The website is www.thehotline.org/ and the phone number is 1-800-799-SAFE.

- Think of the people in your life who always make you feel energized, validated, and happy. Make it a point to spend more time with them!

18. Practice Imperfection

All-or-nothing, perfectionist thinking can obstruct a healthy lifestyle change plan. One technique for breaking this unhealthy thinking pattern is to plan and practice imperfection. For every habit in this book that you choose to try, have a barely-meets-the-requirements version—something completely, utterly imperfect.

Check out bestselling author Stephen Guise's books *Mini Habits* and *Mini Habits for Weight Loss*, as well as *How to Be an Imperfectionist*. These books were inspired by his resolution to work out every day, with the initial workout being one pushup a day. Just one. Consistently doing just one pushup a day eventually brought him robust fitness, as well as a couple of multimillion-copy bestselling books. Being imperfect can lead to some amazing accomplishments.

These teensy little barely habits will bridge you through tough, busy, or lazy times until you can pick up your efforts again. These are placeholder habits that just keep the habit alive.

Tips to Make the Habit Stick

- What's the smallest, teensiest workout that you could manage every single day no matter what? If it's just a toe-touch stretch, then that's perfect.
- Trying to keep a diary? Write: "Crap day today," end of entry.
- Planning to meditate daily? Close your eyes and meditate—for 10 seconds. Yup.
- If it's the Relaxation Response deep breathing technique you want to incorporate, take one deep breath. Just one.
- Remember that these utterly imperfect versions of your ideal habit count and will carry you through the tough times.

Rest Up: Sleep Habits for Your Heart

Getting enough sleep and making it quality sleep are very important pieces of the self-care puzzle. Sleep deprivation triggers the stress response, releasing stress hormones that cause increased heart rate, blood pressure, and fat storage, and has directly negative effects on heart health as well.

19. Create a Consistent Sleep/Wake Schedule

One of the first pieces of advice you will hear from a sleep expert is to maintain a regular sleeping and waking schedule. That means going to bed and waking up at about the same times every day and allowing about 8 hours (more or less, depending on the individual) for sleep. For people who suffer from insomnia, this is critical advice. As a matter of fact, experts advise people with insomnia to wake up (and get up) at the usual early hour even after a night of poor sleep, as this will build up a sleep deficit. This deficit will then help the sleepy person fall asleep faster and sleep better the next night. And yes, that means no napping. The point is to create a consistent schedule, and sleeping in or napping will ruin those efforts. Using medications for sleep is highly unadvised, as these do not address underlying issues and can create dependence. (Using medications to treat other medical problems that can impact sleep, like depression and anxiety, is appropriate. Those issues should be addressed separately.)

So let's figure out your schedule. You can't get enough sleep if you're getting to bed too late. What would be a reasonable bedtime for you? Be honest with yourself: are there any time-wasting activities keeping you up late? Think about how these things may be impacting your health. Is there anything at all helpful about these activities? If so, try to move them up or reduce the time spent so that you can get some much-needed zzz's. If not, think about letting them go so you can get to sleep.

You are unlikely to sleep well if you wake up (and get up) at different times on different days. Set an alarm and get in the habit of getting up and starting your day at the same time, no matter what.

Tips to Make the Habit Stick

- Decide on a reasonable bedtime for yourself. Have you thought of setting an alarm for bedtime? If you tend to go to bed later than you need to, you may want to set that alarm.

- If you're struggling to follow your bedtime schedule, think about what tends to keep you up late. Is it working late into the night? There may be ways to fit work in during daytime hours (while you're at the office). Is it surfing the web, scrolling through social media, or watching TV? See Habit #21.

- How much time do you need to sleep? Not everyone needs 8 hours. Some people need more, some less. Think about how much sleep you need in order to feel refreshed, and set your awake alarm at the appropriate time.

- Set your awake alarm every night and wake up at the same time every morning. Sleeping in (or napping) can interfere with the normal sleep cycle and create sleep problems.

- If you are struggling with insomnia, ask for a referral to a sleep expert. The most effective treatment is cognitive behavioral therapy for insomnia (CBT-I for short), not sleep medications.

- If you think that your sleep issue is related to an underlying medical problem, please talk to a healthcare provider.

20. Create a Consistent (and Clean) Bedtime Routine

Having a consistent and calming bedtime routine can help you get to sleep faster and sleep better. It may take a while to figure out what will work well for you, so be prepared for a little trial and error. Aim for a 15- to 30-minute routine of gentle, quiet activity that will ease you into slumber. It's a good idea to have a bare-minimum version of your routine for busier times. Even if it's only touching your toes and breathing deeply, it will bridge you through busy times so you don't lose the habit.

Tips to Make the Habit Stick

- A cup of tea may help. Chamomile and mint are relaxing. Ginger is excellent for digestion. Valerian root is stinky but sedating.
- Stretching or yoga helps relax the body. This can be done on the floor by the bed, on a rug or a yoga mat.
- Meditation is also helpful, either on your own or using an app or CD that guides you.
- Calming music soothes stress and can ease you into sleep.
- Reading a book or a magazine is allowed, provided you can put it down when you need to.
- Many people pray at bedtime, and this can be an ideal time to practice thankfulness and forgiveness. (Remember Habits #8 and #12?)

21. Say No to Screens

The blue light from screens (phones, computers, TV) can interfere with sleep onset. Not only that, but it can be difficult to put the electronics down once we pick them up. Make it a habit to ban electronics at bedtime. Think about your calming bedtime routine and make time for that instead.

Tips to Make the Habit Stick

- If you're having trouble turning off the electronics, make it harder for yourself to use them. There are apps you can use to "lock" yourself out of social media at certain times. See also Habit #99 ("Make It Harder to Use Your Device") and Habit #100 ("Take Advantage of Technology to Control Your Technology").
- Is there a TV in your bedroom? Remove it. The bedroom is the absolute worst place for a TV.
- Been wanting to read more good books? Here's your chance. Screens are bad, but old-fashioned books are great for bedtime. Pick books that you won't want to stay up all night reading, though.

Team Effort:
Social Support Habits for Your Heart

It's well known that loneliness is associated with depression as well as premature death. In addition, social connection is a key factor for better stress management.

22. Eat with Others

Studies show that when we sit down and eat with others, we eat slower and better. When families eat together, children learn to regulate their food intake, and everyone tends to make healthier choices. When elderly people eat with others, they eat a wider variety of foods and have a significantly lower risk of depression. Overall, people who eat meals with others tend toward a healthier body weight.

This makes intuitive sense. Human beings are social creatures, and we evolved within tribes and villages. It's natural for us to eat in the company of others. Modern life makes communal meals less likely; some people work far from where they live and get home late for dinner. Kids' activities can extend into the evening. Many elderly folks live alone. But making eating with others a priority (plus a little planning) can bring the communal meal—and healthier eating patterns—back into your life.

Tips to Make the Habit Stick

- If you live alone, plan meals with friends. I know one group that rotates weekends, taking turns hosting meals. Even once a month is beneficial, as this builds community and connectedness as well.
- If you have kids, schedule family dinners as often as possible. This is a win-win situation for everyone, and it's well worth the effort.
- If you can, have elderly relatives over for a meal on a regular basis. Are they in a nursing home? Go to them. Bringing the generations together around a meal helps everyone by increasing the quality of the food, slowing the rate of eating, and creating intergenerational connection.
- Make eating together easy. If you cook a big meal, cook extra and freeze it for later. This way, when everyone's running around and gets home late, you can heat it up, and everyone can still sit down together to enjoy it.

23. Nurture Your Best Relationships

People can feel lonely and isolated even when they're surrounded by others. It can be difficult to form close relationships, and, even then, not all relationships are healthy. Identify a couple of people in your life who are stable and supportive. They may be close by or far away. Regardless, if you nurture these relationships, these folks will be more likely to help you when you need it. Maybe they can listen to you vent or offer advice. Just knowing that you have people you can trust who will listen to you when you need them is important.

Tips to Make the Habit Stick

- Think of the people in your life who are stable and supportive. Try to remember their birthdays, congratulate their achievements (or their kids' achievements), send condolence cards when they lose a loved one... Maybe it's just an email or a Facebook message, but recognizing their life events in these small ways means a lot and makes it more likely that they will remember you when you need it.

- If one of these folks reaches out to you when she has a problem, listen to her and offer emotional support. It can be as simple as saying, "I hear what you're saying; that must be hard," or "I'm so sorry you're going through that." She'll be more likely to listen to you when you need her.

- If one of these people invites you to a gathering, be it a work outing or a wedding or a birthday party, try to attend. It can be inconvenient, but if it's not impossible, he will likely appreciate your effort and will be more likely to return the favor when you need people around you.

24. Join a Group

If you don't live near friends and family and you don't know your neighbors, consider joining a group that meets regularly. This can be church/temple/mosque, yoga or other exercise class, a knitting group or book club, or even Alcoholics Anonymous; they all provide a sense of togetherness. Religious communities typically will organize around a member who is having a hard time. They may help a member get to doctor's appointments or even just meet him for coffee and a chat.

Tips to Make the Habit Stick

- If there is an activity you enjoy at a gym or yoga studio, consider signing up. Many people have a particular class they like to attend, and that can be a way to get to know others with similar interests.
- Check out *Meetup* at www.meetup.com/, a website that helps people form and connect to all sorts of recreational groups. A quick perusal of local offerings turns up a trashy romance novels book club, an om chanting meditation group, and "Silver Foxes Martial Arts." I have no doubt that you can find a few groups to suit your tastes.
- If you can identify at all with any religion, consider joining a congregation. Within each faith, there is a very wide spectrum of observance. Whether you strongly identify with religious tenets or prefer a more laid-back and loosely interpreted approach, there is a group out there for you.

25. Use Technology to Connect

Studies show that the quality of relationships is more important than just having relationships, which makes perfect sense. Feeling connected and supported is what's important. If you're far from your friends and family, you can use technology to feel warmth and support. FaceTime and Skype are ways to directly connect with family and friends, but phone calls, emails, and social media can help as well.

This can be especially true if you're going through something that the people around you can't identify with. Maybe it's a particular illness or disease you or a loved one has been diagnosed with or a difficult experience not many other people have been through. Online support groups of all kinds can help you connect with like-minded people.

Tips to Make the Habit Stick

- If you have family far away, stay in touch as much as you can.
- Use social media wisely. Facebook and other sites can be a wonderful way to stay connected, if you're using them to connect. Scrolling through your feed mindlessly is not connecting. Writing someone a meaningful birthday wish or note of support is. Reach out in positive ways.
- If no one can relate to what you're going through, do an Internet search for online support groups or ask around for in-person support groups. If it's a particular diagnosis you or a loved one is dealing with, the medical team can help you identify a foundation or support group. Many patients are willing to be contacted by newly diagnosed individuals who are seeking guidance. This is especially true for rare diseases and certain cancers. Ask your medical team.

26. Live in a Community

If you can, live somewhere where you can know your neighbors and/or live close to friends and family. If you're at a point in your life where you can choose where to live, think about the years ahead and the importance of a solid support network. A high salary or a prestigious job isn't worth much if you're miserable. If children are in your future, and you have family who are able and willing to help care for a child, keep that in mind. No one will care for your child like your family will—especially during difficult times, like unforeseen emergencies and illness. You'll save yourself endless headaches and thousands of dollars. That's a win-win.

There's also the importance of knowing your neighbors. The people who live around you can be an important safety net. Being able to interact with them easily can make relationship-building easier as well. These are the folks who can watch your place when you're away, pick up packages from your front door, or call the police if there's an emergency… And in addition you can enjoy social events like dinners or impromptu over-the-fence chats. Neighbors offer practical connections that also combat loneliness and protect against stress.

Tips to Make the Habit Stick

- Nurture your support network. Check in with folks. Send birthday greetings, congratulate achievements, and attend important functions. These are the people who will help you in times of need, more so if you're a part of their lives. Being engaged with people also makes it easier for you to ask for their help when you need it.
- Take the little opportunities to get to know your neighbors. If you happen to see someone, wave and say, "Hey, how are you?" If you see someone struggling with the trash or a heavy package, offer

to help if you're able. This is especially important if it's someone you're not sure you like very much, but you don't know very well. Negative neighbor impressions often transform into supportive relationships when people get to know one another.

- Give to receive, but don't expect to receive. If your smiles are met with scowls, don't take it personally. If the friendly birthday and holiday greetings you send to a family member or friend are met with silence, don't take offense. As long as a person is not toxic or harmful to you, give her the benefit of the doubt. She may be going through a tough time, and your positive outreach may be very meaningful to her. You never know.

You now have twenty-six Foundational Habits addressing stress, sleep, and social support that will boost your behavioral change plan.

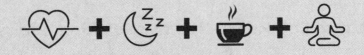

Chapter 5

Eat for Your Life: Nutrition Habits

FOOD IS POWERFUL medicine. My patients who have successfully turned their lives around get the big picture: "diets" don't work; sustainable healthy eating habits do. What we're aiming for is a healthy diet that can be maintained for life.

In this chapter I'll outline twenty-two heart-healthy diet habits and the science behind them, plus specific action advice and delicious recipe suggestions. The recipes, which are provided at the end of the book, were developed with input from a chef and are designed to be scrumptious, simple, flexible, and budget-minded. Making the best food choices can become easy and natural...in other words, habit.

What to Eat: Heart-Healthy Nutrition Habits

This first section is heavy on the nutrition recommendations and the solid science behind them.

27. Aim for Eight Servings of Fruits and Vegetables Per Day (4 to 5 Cups)

There are mountains of scientific studies showing that the more fruits and vegetables we eat, the lower our risk for developing heart disease. Eating more fruits and vegetables can also help prevent heart attacks, strokes, and heart-related deaths in people who are at high risk. According to recent data, 1.7 million deaths per year (including 11 percent of coronary heart disease and 9 percent of stroke deaths) could be prevented if people ate more fruits and vegetables. This is why the World Health Organization and the American Heart Association recommend eight servings (about 4 or 5 cups) of fruits and vegetables daily. Some researchers suggest aiming for ten—yes, ten!—servings of fruits and veggies per day. An analysis of almost one hundred studies and more than two hundred thousand participants found that eating ten servings (about 8 cups) of fruits and vegetables a day was associated with significantly lower risks of premature death from any cause (31 percent), as well as heart disease (24 percent) and stroke (33 percent). Can't do that much? Even two and a half servings of fruits and vegetables per day (about 1½ cups) had some benefits.

So start with at least two and a half, aim for eight, and ideally consume ten servings of fruits and vegetables daily.

Here's where my doctor advice comes in. Many guidelines include fruit juice as "fruit." Science (and logic) begs to differ: fruit juice does not count as fruit.

If counting servings is too cumbersome, then use this visual aid: Picture a plate. If your daily food intake sits on that plate, then ideally, at least half of it will be all fruits and veggies. For an image of this, check out the Harvard School of Public Health's "Healthy Eating Plate" at www.hsph.harvard.edu/nutritionsource/healthy-eating-plate/ or the USDA's MyPlate at www.choosemyplate.gov.

What Does a Serving of Fruits or Vegetables Look Like?

Per the American Heart Association:

Fruits

Whole fresh fruit = 1 piece approximately the size of a baseball. Examples are 1 apple, 1 peach, 1 orange, ½ a banana.

Fresh, frozen, or canned fruit (unsweetened) = ½ cup. Examples are berries, diced peaches, pineapple, mango.

Dried fruit = ¼ cup. Examples are raisins, cherries, dates.

Vegetables

Raw leafy vegetables = 1 cup. Examples are lettuces, kale.

Fresh, frozen, or canned vegetables = ½ cup. Examples are chopped vegetables, unseasoned plain frozen vegetables, and cooked beans.

Based on this, eight servings of fruits and vegetables could look like:

Breakfast: 1 cup of berries

Lunch: 2 cups of lettuce + ½ cup tomatoes + ½ cup cucumbers + an orange for dessert

If you wanted to get to ten servings, then add:

Dinner: 1 cup broccoli + ½ cup diced peppers + ½ cup snow peas (in a stir fry)

Tips to Make the Habit Stick

- Start with at least one serving of fruits and/or vegetables with every meal and snack, and increase over time to two or three. You'll be up to ten in a matter of weeks!
- It's fine to use frozen fruits and vegetables. High-quality berries, tropical fruits, and mixed vegetables are cheaper than fresh and can be bought in bulk from the grocery store and stored in the freezer for long periods.
- Make breakfast with two (or more) servings of fruits and/or veggies. This gets the good stuff in early in the day. Try Filling Fruit and Nut Bowl with Greek Yogurt in Appendix A.
- Free meal tracker apps like MyFitnessPal or Dr. Michael Greger's Daily Dozen app can help you get your ten servings of fruits and veggies daily.

Fresh Local Produce Delivered

You may have heard of community-supported agriculture (CSA), where you pay a membership fee to a local farm and have fresh local produce delivered to your home. This is a terrific way to stock up on produce, and it's less expensive than the grocery store and supports your local farmers. The USDA has a directory of CSAs on its website.

28. Eat More Colorful and Cruciferous Plants

Particularly healthy for your heart are colorful fruits and vegetables (red, orange, yellow, green, blue, and purple), as well as cruciferous vegetables (such as broccoli and cauliflower). These contain natural plant nutrients (like antioxidants) that neutralize toxins and lower inflammation in the body, protecting and healing our arteries and heart. These plant nutrients include carotenoids, flavonoids, glucosinolates, resveratrol, nitrates, and omega-3 fatty acids, as well as vitamins and minerals, fiber, and more. Plant nutrients can't be extracted from plants and stuffed into a pill or capsule, despite the multibillion-dollar health supplement industry's claims. Science says eat the plant. Studies have shown that the more colorful varieties of fruits and vegetables and cruciferous vegetables we eat, the lower our risk of all kinds of cardiovascular disease (including coronary heart disease, heart attacks, strokes, and microvascular disease).

Here is a rainbow of examples of these heart-healthy plant foods:

- **Red:** apples, grapes, peppers, tomatoes, strawberries, raspberries, cranberries
- **Orange:** pumpkins, butternut squash, carrots, sweet potatoes, apricots
- **Yellow:** spaghetti squash, peppers, tomatoes
- **Green:** spinach, collard greens, chard, lettuce (the greener the better)
- **Blue:** blueberries, elderberries, plums, figs
- **Purple:** grapes, cabbage, peppers, carrots, blackberries
- **Cruciferous vegetables:** broccoli, cauliflower, Brussels sprouts, kale, cabbage, mustard and turnip greens

White veggies are good for you as well! Cauliflower, onions, garlic, white potatoes, and tofu all contain important plant nutrients too.

Tips to Make the Habit Stick

- Try new varieties of fruits and vegetables every week. When you shop, pick up something new.
- Aim to have at least three different colors of plants on your plate at every meal.
- Don't like the slightly bitter taste of some veggies, like Brussels sprouts, broccoli, or cauliflower? Try roasting them, which brings out their natural (and good-for-you) sweetness.
- Consider subscribing to a healthy food magazine or look at recipes on apps such as Pinterest for colorful and cruciferous plant recipe ideas. Or try these recipes: Filling Fruit and Nut Bowl with Greek Yogurt, Superfood Lentil Soup, or Super-Simple Cashew Stir-Fry (all in Appendix A).

All Plants Are Superfoods Because They're Full of Nutrients

There are thousands of nutrients in plants, and it's increasingly unlikely that we will ever be able to isolate and package each "supernutrient" into a pill. Supplements have been shown to be useless, possibly contaminated with toxins, and cost a lot of money. Going overboard on just one food can even be harmful (a daily overabundance of kale is associated with thyroid problems, for example). This is why we do not recommend focusing on one particular food or taking supplements for heart health. It's best to get your plant nutrients from a variety of plants, herbs, and spices.

29. Chew Your Fruits (and Vegetables)

A whole-foods approach for best health means eating the whole fruit or vegetable to get the most nutritional benefit. Fruits and vegetables contain water, natural plant sugars and fibers, and many nutrients. Juicing crushes the fruit or vegetable in order to extract the liquid and sugars but leaves many nutrients and all the healthy fiber behind.

Blending (as in smoothies) is moderately better, but we still tend to drink faster than we chew, which allows us to take in more food (and calories) than maybe we intended. The best solution is to eat the food. Chew the fruits and vegetables, the way nature intended. After all, juicers and blenders are modern inventions, and juices and smoothies are faddish.

Tips to Make the Habit Stick

- Stock up on fruits and vegetables that travel well, like apples, oranges, peaches, plums, baby carrots, or peppers (for slicing).
- Always bring fresh fruits and/or veggies to work, and eat them first when you are hungriest so you get in your servings and in the best form.
- At home, don't hide your beautiful colorful produce. Set a bowl full of gorgeous fruit on your kitchen counter or dining room table. If you can see it, you're more likely to eat it.
- If you bring home melon or pineapple, slice it up and store it in the fridge for easy access. If it's already cut up, you're more likely to eat it.
- Set a platter of fresh sliced fruit out for dessert after dinner. It will likely satisfy cravings for sweets.

30. Aim for Three Servings or More a Day of Whole Grains

Studies show that regular intake of whole grains decreases the risk of diabetes and heart disease. But what are whole grains? These are unrefined grains with all parts intact (bran, germ, and endosperm).

The bran is the fiber-rich outer layer. The germ is full of nutrients, including vitamins, minerals, protein, and healthy fats. The endosperm is empty starchy carbohydrate.

Refined white flour and white rice have had all the good parts removed (the bran and germ) and so are missing all the fiber, protein, healthy fats, vitamins, and minerals. They're just empty starchy endosperm.

It's good to know your flours: "enriched flour" is refined white flour that's had some vitamins added to it after processing. This does not make it healthy. As a matter of fact, enriched flour is absolutely the worst choice for you, as it's immediately converted to sugar in your body. This can be bleached or unbleached or organic, but it's still refined flour with all the good parts removed, i.e., empty starchy endosperm.

One hundred percent whole-grain flours are a much healthier choice of flours. If you're going to have pasta or bread, make sure the label lists "100 percent whole wheat" as the first ingredient and does not list any "enriched flour." It's important to note, however, that while 100 percent whole-grain flours are better than refined white flour, the best choice is the intact, unprocessed grain. The more intact the grains are, the slower the carbohydrates are absorbed by the body, which can help prevent weight gain and diabetes.

The bottom line is to avoid white rice and refined white flour and replace them with brown rice and flours made from whole grains (100 percent whole wheat, quinoa, or others). The best choice, though, is the intact whole grain.

Here are examples of some of the more commonly found intact whole grains:

Corn: Corn can be eaten on the cob; kernels can be steamed or roasted; popcorn can be popped (air-popped or with minimal oil). Masa, the fortified flour made from corn and used to make tortillas, counts as a whole-grain flour.

Oats: Yes, oats are a whole grain! The less processed the oats, the better they are for you. So whole oats (also called *groats*) are better than steel-cut oats, which are better than regular oats, which are better than quick-cooking oats. But they all count as whole grains.

Brown rice: Brown rice is real rice that hasn't had the germ and bran removed. This is always better than white rice.

Quinoa: This tiny fast-cooking grain is boiled and then served. It makes a wonderful addition to salads or replacement for white rice.

Farro: This is the whole intact wheat grain berry. It cooks up just like pasta, though it can take 20–30 minutes. Then it's drained and served.

Bulgur: This is cracked wheat, made by cooking, drying, then chopping up the whole-wheat kernels. It's very fast and easy to prepare, and is commonly used in Middle Eastern cooking.

The nonprofit consumer advocacy group Whole Grains Council lists more types of whole grains, along with loads of helpful information and recipes: https://wholegrainscouncil.org/whole-grains-101.

What Does a Serving of Whole Grains Look Like?

Per the American Heart Association:

Intact Whole Grains

½ cup cooked corn, oats, brown rice, quinoa, farro*, bulgur*, amaranth, millet

3 cups unsalted, air-popped popcorn

Whole-Grain Products

½ cup whole-wheat pasta*

1 slice whole-grain bread (such as 100 percent whole-wheat bread)*

1 (6-inch) whole-wheat* or corn tortilla

5 whole-grain crackers*

1 cup ready-to-eat, whole-grain cold cereal*

(*These contain gluten.)

Tips to Make the Habit Stick

- If you're going to eat bread or pasta, always buy 100 percent whole wheat and check the label to ensure there's no "enriched" wheat flour added.

- Consider buying grains in bulk. It's cheaper. Even better: order whole grains in bulk from an online source (like www.nuts.com) and have them delivered right to your home.

- When you prepare whole grains for a recipe, make more than you need and freeze in portion-sized bags for the next recipe. This works very well with brown rice, quinoa, and farro.

- Adding whole grains to a salad makes it a meal! Try these easy salads: Nutty Tabbouleh Salad; Summer Corn, Tomato, Spinach, and Basil Salad (in Appendix A).

31. Have Some Fiber-Rich Foods Every Day (Especially Legumes!)

The American Heart Association recommends about 30 grams of dietary fiber per day for the average person (based on a 2,000 calorie/day diet). But what is dietary fiber, and how do we know how many grams we're getting?

Dietary fiber, also known as *roughage*, is a carbohydrate found in plants. We can't absorb fiber, yet it has many beneficial health effects. There are two kinds, soluble or insoluble, and both are good for us. In our intestines, soluble fiber becomes a thick gel that traps fats so they can't be absorbed, which lowers cholesterol levels and slows digestion, which in turn keeps blood sugars from spiking. Good sources include oatmeal, beans, lentils, and many fruits. Insoluble fiber helps keep our stools regular and soft; good sources include whole grains, beans, lentils, and many vegetables. Both make us feel full, which helps us eat less.

Many of these fiber-rich foods are a part of the Mediterranean diet, which is long associated with lower risk of heart disease. Legumes, which include beans, lentils, and peas, are a staple of the Mediterranean diet and are particularly rich in both soluble and insoluble fiber and are also a fantastic source of plant protein and nutrients. A cup of cooked garbanzo beans has about 14 grams of protein as well as 12 grams of fiber. These beans are a great source of folate, iron, magnesium, vitamin A, and calcium. People who eat legumes daily are more likely to have a smaller waistline and are less likely to be overweight or obese, or to develop diabetes or metabolic syndrome. Basically, legumes are really good for you in many ways, but especially for your heart.

Tips to Make the Habit Stick

- Add beans to a salad for a boost of heart and gastrointestinal nutrition. They count as both protein and fiber.
- No time? It's fine to use canned. Choose unsalted or if the fruits, vegetables, or legumes have salt, rinse them in running water (rinsing can remove up to half of the added salt). Or try quick-cooking red lentils, which can be ready to eat in less than 10 minutes.
- If you're going to make the longer-cooking versions, make extra and freeze some for another meal. They thaw perfectly and can be easily added to soups or salads.
- If you're not used to eating a lot of fiber, then start with a little and increase over time. This will minimize gas and bloating, and your body will adjust if you keep it up.
- When you're increasing the amount of fiber you eat, you also need to increase the amount of water you drink. Fiber soaks up fluids (think sawdust on a barroom floor...). If there isn't enough water in your intestines, fiber won't pass through very well, which can lead to constipation. Hydrate!
- Try these recipes: Overnight Oats; Superfood Lentil Soup; Antioxidant Chili (in Appendix A).

32. Get Some Omega-3s Every Day

Here's where we get into the heart-healthy fats. Unsaturated fats are healthy, and these can be monounsaturated or polyunsaturated (PUFAs). Certain PUFAs, the omega-3 fats DHA (docosahexaenoic acid), EPA (eicosapentaenoic acid), and ALA (alpha-linolenic acid), are associated with a significantly lower risk of heart and related diseases, and it's recommended to increase the amount of these in our diet. DHA and EPA are found mainly in seafood, while ALA is found mainly in plants (though our liver does convert some ALA into EPA and DHA). Regular intake of a small amount (approximately 200 mg) of omega-3 fats daily is associated with a significantly lower risk of heart and related diseases. This effect has primarily been seen with food sources, not supplements.

You may have also read about other PUFAs, the omega-6 fats. Though some research suggests that these are not as healthy as omega-3 fats, they are a heck of a lot healthier than most saturated fats and trans fats, and it's not worth fretting over.

Tips to Make the Habit Stick

- If you're in the habit of eating meats like beef, chicken, and pork, try switching some of those meals to seafood instead.
- Fresh seafood can be expensive. Many canned varieties provide the same health benefits but at a far lower price. Good for your heart and your budget!
- Try these recipes: Niçoise-Style Sardine Salad and Secret Ingredient Baltimore-Style Salmon Patties with Not-Oily Aioli (in Appendix A).
- Research does not show a benefit to taking omega-3 supplements (such as fish oil and krill oil). Supplements can be contaminated

with toxins and are expensive. It's better to get your omega-3 fats in your food.

- People who do not or cannot eat fish can get plenty of omega-3 fats through other food sources. The ALA in plants has health benefits, and some is converted to DHA and EPA in our body. Walnuts, flax and chia seeds, and edamame (soybeans) are excellent food sources of ALA.
- Try the Apple Cinnamon Walnut Overnight Oats recipe in Appendix A.

33. Choose Healthier Fats

There has been some controversy over fats in the news, with headlines declaring "Butter Is Back," citing studies that showed no difference between saturated and unsaturated fats for heart disease risk. Here's the problem with that research: years ago when low-fat foods hit the market, companies had to do something to make the foods taste good, so they added sugar. A lot of sugar. People who ate these low-saturated-fat foods still got heart disease, and butter didn't look like the bad guy. The science community howled in outrage over the unhealthy misconceptions being spread around, hitting back with headlines like "No, Butter Is Not Back: Eat in Moderation, Please." Research backs this up. A study of fifty-nine thousand participants at risk for heart disease found that when saturated fat was replaced with sugars, there was no heart benefit. When saturated fat was replaced by polyunsaturated fats, there was a 17 percent lower risk of heart attacks and sudden cardiac death.

When we directly compare saturated versus unsaturated fats, things are much clearer. High-quality research looking at more than thirteen thousand participants with risk factors for heart disease found that when saturated fats were replaced with polyunsaturated fats, there was a 19 percent lower risk of having a heart attack or sudden cardiac death. Another study followed more than seven thousand participants with significant risk for heart disease over a period of five years. Participants were given either the Mediterranean diet plus olive oil or nuts or a regular diet. The Mediterranean diet plus olive oil or nuts was associated with a 30 percent lower risk of heart attacks, strokes, or cardiac death compared to the regular diet (and these results stood when the study was reexamined in 2018).

If we add up all the data, it's clear we should aim for healthier polyunsaturated and monounsaturated fats and less of other fats. The best and easiest way to do this is to steer clear of packaged, processed foods and all fast foods. Those are the biggest sources of unhealthy fats in our diets.

What About Cheese, Milk, and Yogurt?

You can safely enjoy these in moderation. Most cheeses, whole milk, and full-fat yogurt contain a fair amount of saturated fat, but they also contain protein and calcium. For those who love their dairy and do not have heart disease, it's fine to enjoy a few servings a week, preferably of naturally higher-protein, lower-fat dairy such as ricotta, fresh mozzarella, feta, milk, and yogurt.

In summary, if we replace the less-healthy and harmful fats in our diet with healthier ones, we can lower our risk for cardiovascular disease (heart attacks, strokes) by 30 percent. That's just as powerful as a cholesterol-lowering medication!

Tips to Make the Habit Stick

- Avoid processed foods, especially processed meats and fast foods.
- Stock up on healthy oils so that you'll have them when you need them. Extra-virgin olive, flaxseed, walnut, almond, canola, corn, sunflower, and safflower oils are fine. Sesame oil is especially useful for flavoring Asian salads or stir-fries. Keep a few in your pantry, ready for recipes.
- Always choose extra-virgin olive oil. Other olive oils, like "light" and "organic," are less healthy because they're made from super-processing the olives or from adding other oils, which may not be unsaturated.

34. Eat Four Servings of Nuts Per Week

Nuts are good for your heart and your life. Research shows that eating four servings of nuts per week was associated with a significantly lower risk of having coronary heart disease (19 percent) or any type of cardiovascular disease (28 percent). There was also a significantly lower risk of dying from coronary heart disease (22 percent), cardiovascular disease (22 percent), sudden cardiac death (75 percent), or anything at all (19 percent). The studies looked at tree nuts (which include almonds, walnuts, pistachios, and hazelnuts) as well as peanuts (which are technically a legume but nutritionally similar to tree nuts).

Another study found that for every one serving per week increase in nuts, there was a 10 percent lower risk of having coronary heart disease. This may be due to the fact that nuts are a rich source of healthy oils. Nuts also are great sources of both soluble and insoluble fiber, as well as vitamins and minerals. Nuts are an important part of the classic Mediterranean diet, which we know is a very good diet for heart health. (Allergies are a consideration here. For people who are allergic to nuts, this habit doesn't apply. As a doctor, I'm going to remind you to update your epinephrine auto-injector and carry it with you at all times!)

What Does One Serving Size of Nuts Look Like?

Per the National Heart, Lung, and Blood Institute (NHLBI):

- $\frac{1}{3}$ cup nuts (equal to $1\frac{1}{2}$ ounces)
- 2 tablespoons nut butter

Tips to Make the Habit Stick

- Regularly stock up on nuts, but keep budget in mind. Nuts are cheaper when bought in larger quantities or ordered online. Shop around for your favorite sources.
- Nuts can go rancid. Store them in airtight containers. Glass is ideal.
- Make a portion of your favorite nuts a regular go-to snack. Have some in your bag or desk at work at all times.
- Get in the habit of adding a handful of nuts to your meals, be it yogurt, oatmeal, salads, or stir-fries.
- Try these recipes: Apple Cinnamon Walnut Overnight Oats; Filling Fruit and Nut Bowl with Greek Yogurt; Nutty Tabbouleh Salad (in Appendix A).

35. Enjoy Two to Three Servings of Dark Chocolate Per Week

Research has consistently shown that people who regularly eat chocolate have lower blood pressure, blood sugars, and less heart disease. Chocolate comes from the toasted seeds of the cacao plant, which is rich in healthy plant chemicals called *flavonoids*, specifically cocoa flavanols. Cocoa flavanols have beneficial effects on our blood vessels by neutralizing toxins, which helps prevent stiffness and plaque buildup, as well as promoting healing.

The darker the chocolate, the more cocoa flavanols it has. Milk chocolate sometimes has barely any (it can range from 10–50 percent) and also tends to have more unhealthy fat added. For this reason, I recommend only dark chocolate (at least 60 percent cacao, though the darker the better) and only a small amount. One serving is two small squares (about 50–60 grams total), and science suggests that two or three servings per week provide the most benefit.

Do you like chocolate, but not dark chocolate? It is less sweet but definitely much better for you than milk chocolate. The intense cocoa taste is what can help prevent us from overeating this calorie-dense treat. Start with a small amount and build up over time. The less milk chocolate you eat, the more dark chocolate will begin to taste like normal chocolate to you.

Tips to Make the Habit Stick

- Add a teaspoon of pure unsweetened cocoa powder to your coffee in the morning for a mocha treat.
- Use only dark chocolate chips or chunks (60 percent or higher cacao) in baking and cooking.

- Try these recipes: Dark Chocolate–Dipped Strawberries; Orange Pistachio Dark Chocolate Bark; Cherry Chocolate Overnight Oats (in Appendix A).
- Use pure unsweetened cocoa powder in your savory cooking as well. Try the Antioxidant Chili recipe in Appendix A.
- If you have a tendency to eat more than a serving (two small squares), consider buying only small amounts at a time or dividing what you buy into serving sizes as soon as you get home.

36. Spice (and Herb) It Up

Fruits and vegetables are not the only excellent sources of plant nutrients. Herbs (parts of leafy green plants used for flavoring or teas) and spices (roots, seeds, berries, or bark used for flavoring or teas) are also rich in these critically important healthy plant chemicals, including antioxidants, vitamins, and minerals. Many of these compounds have been shown to have antibacterial, antiviral, antioxidant, and anti-inflammatory properties. This suggests that they can help prevent or heal damage to the body. However, quality research studies on the health effects of herbs and spices in humans are lacking. Why is that? Well, for one, Big Pharma is not going to fund randomized clinical trials on compounds that are already widely available. No one can patent turmeric, or cinnamon, or ginger, or oregano... Attempts to isolate the "secret ingredient" in these plants, put it in a pill, and see what it does to people (so it can be patented and marketed) have failed to show any significant effects. Basically, there's no profit.

The studies that have been done support using herbs and spices often, but in normal culinary amounts, like in everyday cooking. Promising herbs include chives, dill, thyme, sage, oregano, parsley, marjoram, rosemary, mint, lemongrass, and more. Spices include cinnamon, cloves, cumin, coriander, fennel, mustard, saffron, ginger, bay leaf, fenugreek, turmeric, poppy seed, red chili, and more. (Note: turmeric is especially promising as a powerful antioxidant and anti-inflammatory, but again, the official recommendation is to use everyday spice-aisle turmeric in normal cooking amounts.) I would also mention alliums like garlic and onions (okay, technically not herbs and spices, but they are also plant nutrient-rich and often used in cooking).

Extra herb and spice bonus: research shows that when we add flavorful herbs and spices to our food, we're less likely to add salt (see Habit #39).

Tips to Make the Habit Stick

- Have fun in the spice aisle! Make it a goal to try different spices in your cooking.
- Try tea. Many teas are actually herbs and spices. Drinking a cup of tea in the afternoon or evening is calming, keeps us from snacking, and may provide us with additional benefits.
- Dried herbs and spices can get old and lose their benefits. If yours don't smell fragrant and robust, consider replacing them.
- Grow an herb garden. Indoor herb gardens are widely available; you can order a small one online. Or plant a garden outdoors. Herb gardens are beautiful, fragrant, and provide an inexpensive source of herbs for cooking—much cheaper than buying herbs fresh at the grocery store.
- Buy herbs at farmers' markets. Big bunches are available at far lower prices than at the grocery store. These can be used for tea— yes, fresh herbs can be used as tea—or dried at home for later use.

What Not to Eat: Habits to Avoid Heart-Unhealthy Foods

We've touched on some of these risky foods in Chapter 1. Here's more practical advice for day-to-day healthy habit-forming:

37. Don't Buy or Eat Processed Foods

There is ample high-quality scientific evidence showing a strong link between a diet high in processed foods and an increased risk of heart disease, as well as many other diseases. So we should make it a habit to stay away from processed foods as much as possible. The first step is to recognize processed foods when you see them. These include many foods in plastic packaging or boxes, anything made with bleached or enriched flour, most fast foods, and almost everything in the snack food and cereal aisles.

Not all processed foods are evil, however. Whole-grain pastas, breads, and cereals, and some other foods are fine when included as part of a diet high in plants. Canned, frozen, dried, and baked fruits and veggies may be minimally processed and pure (i.e., without added chemicals or salt).

Look at labels, and if you see an ingredient you cannot pronounce, chances are it is something that has been processed more than you need. Over time, as you grow accustomed to looking at labels and buying fresh foods as much as possible, grocery shopping will be easier and faster.

Tips to Make the Habit Stick

- When you go to the grocery store, buy less food from the middle (the snack food, cereal, and canned food aisles) and more from the outer edges (the produce and seafood sections).
- Look at labels and avoid foods with lots of chemical ingredients.
- Make a rough menu plan for the week or stick to a similar plan week to week. You'll always know what you need from the grocery store, and you'll be less likely to buy junk.
- Decide that you are not a person who eats processed foods and make it a part of your identity.
- Avoid fast foods as much as possible.

38. Limit Meats, Especially Red and Processed Meats

All animal-based products are associated with an increased risk of heart disease and premature death, but not to the same degree. The worst offenders include cured, smoked, and processed meats (like most bacon, sausage, and deli meats). The next is red meat (i.e., beef, veal, pork, lamb). Yes, despite ad campaigns funded by Big Agro, pork is classified as a red meat. The classification is based on the amount of myoglobin, which is the iron-carrying molecule in animals, not the color of the meat. White meats (poultry) follow, though the association with heart disease is far lower. Fish and other seafood, eggs, and dairy are largely without great risk, though the healthiest approach is to consume mostly plants. This is also best for the environment. There is plenty of protein in plant foods, especially beans, lentils, and peas. If you eat animals or animal products, aim for occasional chicken, eggs, seafood, and dairy.

Tips to Make the Habit Stick

- Consider being "vegan before 6," a concept popularized by food journalist and cookbook author Mark Bittman. This means eating vegan for most of the day, then having an omnivorous dinner. I will point out, however, that it is possible to eat vegan and still be eating unhealthily. After all, breads, pastas, and sugars are all technically vegan. Rather, I recommend eating "plant-based before 6."
- Make meat (or fish, or eggs…) the side dish. A really effective strategy is to make your veggies the main attraction of your meal, filling the bulk of your plate. Really we should be aiming for half the plate to be veggies anyways (remember the Healthy Eating Plate visual from Habit #27).

39. Limit High-Sodium Foods (and Salt)

A high-sodium diet is associated with high blood pressure and heart disease. We usually think of sodium and salt as being the same thing. But the table salt we add to our home-cooked food is not usually the culprit. There is sodium in table salt, but it's the sodium in canned and processed foods as well as takeout that is far more likely to cause us problems. Limit the canned and processed foods and takeout in your diet, and you will also be limiting sodium. We should all eat less than 2,300 milligrams (mg) of sodium daily, though less than 1,500 mg daily is healthier. People with high blood pressure or heart conditions should eat even less. To put this in perspective: 1 teaspoon of table salt contains about 2,300 mg of sodium.

Tips to Make the Habit Stick

- Learn how to read food labels for sodium content. Aim for at least under 2,300 mg and ideally under 1,500 mg per day total. (If you have high blood pressure, ask your doctor what your daily limit of sodium is.)
- Canned foods, frozen entrées, and processed and cured meats tend to be highest in sodium in addition to takeout. Limit these foods.
- When you first cut down on sodium, food can taste different for a while. Your taste buds will adjust. Give it some time.
- Try adding more herbs and spices to your foods, which has the added bonus of giving you more detoxifying plant nutrients!

What to Drink: The Best Beverage Habits

What we drink is just as important to our health as what we eat.

40. Hydrate Right

Drink plenty of water throughout the day. There are many reasons. One, it's common to confuse thirst with hunger. Quench thirst first, before reaching for food. Two, we need to take in enough fluid with our food in order to help it pass through our bodies, especially if we're increasing the amount of dietary fiber in our diets. Dehydration can cause constipation. Three, dehydration can also lead to urinary problems, such as urinary tract infections and kidney stones. Fill your glass with water often and flush everything through your system. Four, juices, sodas, and sweetened drinks are loaded with sugars. Drink water or seltzer instead. Tea and coffee are fine; actually, studies show that these contain antioxidants that may promote health (see Habit #41).

Tips to Make the Habit Stick

- Have a water bottle (a reusable one) with you always.
- When you go to a restaurant, always ask for water first before other beverages. Finish your glass before your meal and have more water with your meal.

41. Drink Tea or Coffee Regularly

Both green and black teas are loaded with healthy antioxidants. Both come from the same plants; green tea is minimally processed (steamed and dried), while black tea is lightly fermented. Studies have shown that consuming these teas regularly helps lower blood pressure and improve blood flow. Drink a cup or two of green or black tea daily.

For most people, coffee is also a heart-healthy antioxidant-rich beverage. Drinking about 3 to 4 cups of coffee a day is associated with a lower risk of heart disease or death from heart disease. Coffee is not recommended for pregnant women due to a slightly increased risk of miscarriage, preterm birth, and low-birth-weight babies. Drinking too much coffee or tea can cause anxiety, palpitations, and insomnia from the caffeine. Also keep in mind that if you drown your coffee or tea with cream and sugar or chemicals, you may lose any beneficial effect.

As with everything else, a normal, moderate intake is suggested. One to 2 cups of green or black tea and 3 to 4 cups of coffee seem to be beneficial for the heart (for people who can safely drink these beverages).

Tips to Make the Habit Stick

- An electric kettle at home or work makes tea preparation much easier and faster. Bring your tea bags with you to save money.
- Keep your tea fresh. Tea, just like any other herb or spice, can get old and lose its health benefits.
- Enjoy a cup of tea or coffee in the morning, when it can become part of your morning routine (if it isn't already), but avoid it at bedtime when the caffeine content can keep you awake.
- Have a travel mug or two so that you can brew coffee or tea at home and bring it with you to save money.

42. Limit Alcohol, Although a Small Amount Daily Can Be Heart-Protective

People who drink a small amount of alcohol every day tend to have lower risk of coronary heart disease when compared to people who don't drink or to people who drink heavily. Research shows that light drinking can lower the risk of developing heart disease a great deal (between 40 and 70 percent) and also lower the risk of related diseases such as strokes, aortic aneurysms, and peripheral arterial disease. Wine (red wine especially) seems to be the best choice, though the protective effect is seen with all types of alcohol. The active component in red wine is thought to be an antioxidant plant nutrient called *resveratrol*, but studies that have isolated this compound and given it to participants as a supplement have not shown any promising results to date. (Of note, that seems to be the case with all supplements.)

But this doesn't mean it's advisable to pick up a drinking habit. Alcohol won't erase the risk brought on by other factors. Drinking any amount over what's recommended will actually increase the risk of heart disease by causing high triglycerides (a form of cholesterol), high blood pressure, and weight gain. Alcohol can also be directly toxic to the heart and is associated with arrhythmias like atrial fibrillation. Drinking too much—even just a little too much—also increases the risk of cancer (particularly breast cancer), liver disease, and, obviously, alcohol addiction.

For all of these reasons, the American Heart Association recommends that people do *not* start drinking alcohol as a means to lower their heart disease risk.

For people who can safely drink, and who partake regularly, here is what is recommended:

Men: No more than one to two drinks per day

Women: No more than one drink per day

Definition of a Drink:

- 5 ounces of wine
- 12 ounces of beer
- 1½ ounces of 80-proof spirits
- 1 ounce of 100-proof spirits

Tips to Make the Habit Stick

- Hydrate well before you have any alcohol. If you're thirsty, you may unintentionally drink too much too quickly.
- Measure out your drink (5 ounces of wine, 12 ounces of beer) and then put the bottle or six-pack away.
- If you're having mixed drinks, specify how much hard liquor you want and watch the bartender measure. Some bartenders are a little heavy-handed with the bottle.
- If you're entertaining, mix up a pitcher of a tempting mocktail and have plenty of healthy and delicious appetizers on hand. It's good for you and everyone else as well.
- Try the Bubbly Minty Mojito Mocktail recipe in Appendix A.

How to Shop: Heart-Healthy Grocery Habits

In order to eat healthy for life, we must learn to shop healthy too.

43. Make Your Grocery List Reflect Your Good Food Goals

Plants should make up the bulk of your groceries. Whether fresh/frozen or healthy canned, it's all good. As a matter of fact, fruits and vegetables are typically harvested at their peak of ripeness just prior to being frozen, so they can be an excellent source of vital antioxidants. Buy beans, dry or canned (no-salt is the best). Aim for whole grains: brown rice, oats, quinoa, farro (my favorite), and corn. Yes, remember, corn is a whole grain!

Consider ordering your groceries online. This is a surefire way to avoid being near any unhealthy foods and will help you to always choose healthy foods. If you can, it's a potentially diet-saving option to make a list and order it online for pickup or delivery, rather than expose yourself to all the sights and scents of the grocery store. Even better, support your local farmers by joining a community-supported agriculture (CSA) program.

Tips to Make the Habit Stick

- Use a list when you shop. There are apps you can use so that you can build up your list over a few days.
- Make it easy to order groceries. If you have a grocery app on your phone, you can place your order anytime, like while on the Stair-Master at the gym or on the train.
- Set a regular ordering schedule for your CSA farm delivery. Maybe even put it into your smartphone calendar.

44. Win the Grocery Mind Games

Big business wants to derail your healthy eating plans. They're the ones who invented habit science because they want you to be in the habit of buying their products. But if you know their tricks, you won't fall for them.

For starters, don't go food shopping when you're hungry. Many a well-intentioned healthy eating plan has been derailed by the trip to the grocery store on an empty stomach. If you're starving and you enter the place where all kinds of foods are readily available, you are more likely to make poor choices. Millions of dollars of marketing research have gone into product advertising and placement for exactly this reason. More and more grocery chains also feature restaurants, with a dizzying array of take-out options. In short, if you walk in famished, you'll walk out full. It's a minefield out there, folks. Don't let big business win the grocery games. Stick to your list and ignore their displays. Make sure you've eaten something healthy and satisfying before you go grocery shopping.

Tips to Make the Habit Stick

- Have an apple before you go to the grocery store.
- Always shop with a list and get in the habit of sticking to it.
- Keep a secret stash of portion-sized nut snacks in your backpack or purse. That healthy snack can protect you from giving in to unhealthy temptations.
- See Habit #43: consider ordering groceries online for pickup or delivery and eliminate this issue altogether!

How to Eat: Heart-Healthy Meal Habits

Now you have a lot of suggestions about what to eat and drink and how to grocery shop. Here are some action suggestions for meal preparation and consumption.

45. Make Your Own Well-Balanced Meals

Prepare your own food as much as possible. People who make their own meals tend to eat healthier foods and fewer calories. Restaurant food is typically loaded with extra calories in the form of fat, as well as sodium. In addition, home-cooked meals cost far less than restaurant food.

Make your homemade meals well-balanced. Meals that are high in fiber and complex carbohydrates and include healthy protein and fat can keep you full and satisfied for longer, so you eat less during your day. Fruits and vegetables contain plant nutrients that help protect and heal your blood vessels (Habits #27 and #28). Not only does fiber fill you up, but it is also good for you (remember Habit #31). Healthy fats are also heart-protective (Habits #32 and #33). If you can imagine your food on a plate, use this formula as a guide: your plate should be half (or more) fruits and veggies, a quarter or so whole grains, and a quarter or so lean protein, with some healthy fat.

Tips to Make the Habit Stick

- A well-balanced home-cooked meal does not need to be complicated or fancy. My breakfast takes all of 3 minutes to prepare: 2½ to 3 cups of frozen berries topped with nuts and served alongside a low-sugar yogurt.
- Try these recipes: Superfood Lentil Soup, Antioxidant Chili, or Nutty Tabbouleh Salad (in Appendix A).

46. Make Regular and Recurring Meal Choices

Become a creature of habit when it comes to food. Repeating the same rotation of healthy meal choices over and over helps reinforce them. The fewer things you have to choose between, the less you have to think about them. If your meal choices rarely vary, then even when you're at a restaurant or traveling, your eyes will seek out similar items on any menu: fruit, nuts, yogurt; salads and seafood; healthy soups and snacks. You're less likely to get sidetracked by unhealthy offerings.

Think about your usual day and when you want (and don't want) to eat, and then create a reasonable eating schedule. Studies show that people with a stable eating pattern are better able to maintain a healthy weight. The schedule helps you eat when you're supposed to and not eat when you're not supposed to, so you will be less likely to snack. This is particularly key for work settings, where tempting treats may be sitting around.

Tips to Make the Habit Stick

- Cultivate a list of your favorite meals and rotate these throughout the week. As time goes on, your favorite meals will become easier and easier to shop for and prepare, which will further reinforce your healthy eating habits.
- Establish a regular meal and snack schedule. It doesn't have to be the same every day. For many people their workweek schedule will differ from their weekend schedule. That's okay—just have an idea of what your schedule will be and stick to it.
- Apps such as MyFitnessPal and SparkPeople help you keep your meal choices and schedule on track and are free.

47. Sit Down and Slow Down

People who eat while driving, walking, working at their desk, or watching TV tend to eat more. Studies show that when we sit down to eat, we eat more slowly, make better food choices, and tend to eat less. Sit at a table, spread out your food, and enjoy. Being mindful and present when you eat will help you eat better.

Tips to Make the Habit Stick

- Always sit down to eat, ideally with other people.
- Try not to eat at your work desk.
- Definitely don't eat in your car.
- Make it a habit never to eat in front of a screen. That means the computer, TV, and movies. (Seriously, when was the last time you ate something healthy at the movie theater?)

48. Brush Your Teeth After Every Meal

Dental habits are very important for heart heath. There is a link between poor dental hygiene and gum disease to heart and related diseases. Scientists think this is because bacteria in the gums trigger inflammation throughout the body. Inflammation in the blood promotes arterial plaque and atherosclerosis. Your dental hygienist who encourages you to brush effectively and floss consistently is supporting your heart and your dental health!

Tips to Make the Habit Stick

- Bring a toothbrush and toothpaste to work and make it a habit to brush after eating. This also has the bonus of fresh breath.
- Bring a toothbrush and toothpaste when you'll be out and about for the day or while traveling. It's more and more common to see people brushing in public restrooms. Inspire others!
- Brushing and flossing after a meal is not only good for your gums, but it also helps signal the end of eating. You're less likely to continue eating if you just made the effort to clean your teeth.

Putting It All Together

When you put all of these recommendations together, you get an evidence-based, doctor-approved eating plan: a heart-healthy, well-balanced, varied, and interesting diet made up of fruits and vegetables, whole grains, legumes, maybe some seafood, chicken and eggs, low-fat dairy, herbs and spices, and healthy fats, with plenty of water, some tea and coffee, and maybe some red wine. This will give you all the plant nutrients, healthy complex carbohydrates, dietary fiber, unsaturated fats, lean protein, and fluids you need and will be heart-protective. In addition, you'll be avoiding processed foods such as refined grains, added sugars and chemicals, saturated and trans fats, unhealthy meats and meat products, or too much of anything. You have recommendations to plan, shop, prepare for, and cook consistently balanced and enjoyably mindful meals. You also have the suggestions and recipes to make these recommendations your daily habits.

For best results pick one or a couple habits and try them out. All are doable and can be adjusted to your own life. If you're struggling, look at the suggestions in Chapter 3. Think about why you're getting derailed and use the strategies presented to get yourself back on track. If you're really struggling, ask for help from a healthcare provider or mental health professional.

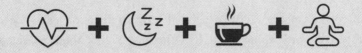

Chapter 6

Lose Weight for Good: Healthy Weight Loss Habits

IF YOU HAVE weight to lose, losing it will lower your risk for heart disease. And it doesn't have to be a lot. Shaving off only 5 percent of total body weight is significant. An analysis of fifty-four studies including more than thirty thousand people with obesity showed that those who completed yearlong diet and exercise-based weight loss programs reduced their risk of death from any cause by 18 percent. Here's what's so amazing: the average weight loss was only 7½ pounds!

Lifestyle change is an amazingly effective strategy for losing weight and especially for keeping it off. That's because it's not about going on a diet or joining the gym. It's about changing your approach to food and exercise so that a healthy diet and active lifestyle become natural. What you eat and what you do has to feel good so you can keep it up and want to keep it up. That way, your healthy lifestyle will become habit.

What to Eat: Nutrition Habits for Healthy Weight Loss

The best part of weight loss counseling is telling people about all the things they can and should eat!

49. Eat More! Fill Up with Fruits and Vegetables

You'll be happy to learn that the first rule of healthy weight loss is to eat more. More plants, that is. The fiber will fill you, and the nutrition will heal you. Fruits and vegetables should make up most of your daily food intake. If you're eating a variety of colorful plants, you do not need to worry much about portions. No one gained weight from eating apples, broccoli, and carrots. Or watermelon, for that matter.

Note that this is not true for blended or juiced fruits and vegetables. Blending and drinking make it easier to take in more food, and more quickly. We tend to consume more in a smoothie than we would have if we'd just eaten the foods whole, and we tend to do so a lot faster, which can make our blood sugar spike as well. And juicing? This not only causes our blood sugar to spike even higher, but it also removes most of what makes fruits and vegetables good for you in the first place. The best way to eat fruits and vegetables is to just eat them, whole or sliced or chopped or cooked.

And as we learned from Chapter 5, consuming eight servings (4 to 5 cups) of fruits and vegetables per day significantly lowers risk of heart disease and stroke, and ten servings per day (about 8 cups) is even better! Remember, juice never counts as a serving of fruits and vegetables.

Tips to Make the Habit Stick

- Have fruits and vegetables with every meal and snack. Ideally you should have them first. An apple before going out to dinner gets a serving of fruit in and helps fill you up so that you eat less overall. A salad at the restaurant can do the same. Making dinner for friends? Set out beautiful platters of colorful roasted vegetables, light corn chips, and sliced veggies with healthy salsa or bean dip, and munch away without guilt.
- Try the Almost Homemade Corn Tortilla Chips with Black Bean Salsamole recipe in Appendix A.
- Remember, frozen and canned fruits and veggies count (as long as there isn't added sugar or salt). Frozen and canned goods are a great way to try new foods and recipes without risking rotted produce. We've all bought beautiful produce and then never found time to make the recipe. If it's safe in the freezer or pantry, that won't happen. Also, it'll be there when you need it for a quick meal on short notice.

50. You Don't Have to Eat Breakfast, But Make Your First Meal a Healthy One

When you're not hungry, your body is trying to tell you something: that you're not hungry. If you're trying to lose weight, listen to your body. This is especially true for breakfast, despite popular belief. Yes, studies of people who have lost and maintained their weight loss show that they tend to eat breakfast in the mornings. But look closer: this is probably more related to their healthy routine, sticking to a schedule, and eating during the daytime (and not close to bedtime) than to eating first thing in the morning. That advice to eat breakfast "to get the metabolism going" is a myth. If you're not hungry first thing in the morning, don't eat. It's fine and will help your body burn fat stores. (For more on this, see Habit #74, "Consider Intermittent Fasting.")

Whenever or whatever your first meal of the day is, make it healthy.

Tips to Make the Habit Stick

- Create a small menu of regular "first meal of the day" choices. The more you repeat the same healthy meal over and over, the less you have to think about it, and the more likely it is to become habit.

- Note that barely any acceptable breakfast options come from the cereal aisle or the bakery. Traditional breakfast foods are laden with refined flours, added sugar, and saturated fat. The healthy breakfast recipes in this book can be enjoyed at any time of the day!

- Our body doesn't require much food for optimal health, but it does require fluids. If you're skipping a meal, remember to hydrate with water, seltzer, coffee or tea, but not juice.

51. Balance Your Salad

"Oh, I'll just order a salad," sounds very healthy, but if it's a typical Cobb salad, Chinese chicken salad, or a loaded wedge salad, then it's not. And if it's a small side salad (which is usually served on a little plate you could use to feed a rabbit), then it may not hold you over, and you'll be searching for a vending machine later. If you're going to eat a salad, make it healthy and satisfying with plenty of plant nutrients, fiber, protein, and healthy fats. This will prevent your blood sugar from spiking, keep you feeling full for longer, and protect your heart. A basic formula for a well-balanced salad is:

- **The base:** This can be greens (lettuce, spinach, kale, collard greens, chard, cabbage) or vegetables (broccoli and cauliflower).
- **The mix-ins:** This can be any assortment of colorful raw or roasted vegetables (chopped tomatoes, peppers, cucumbers, radishes, eggplant, carrots) or even fruits (apples, berries).
- **The protein:** This can be plant-based, like beans (kidney, garbanzo, white, navy, black), lentils (any color), peas, tofu; or animal-based, like shrimp, fish (ideally cold-water fatty fish like salmon [canned is fine]), or broiled/grilled/poached chicken.
- **The topping:** Good sources of healthy fats and proteins include nuts (sliced almonds, walnuts, cashews, pine nuts, even peanuts) and seeds (pumpkin, sesame).
- **The dressing:** Ideally you'd use healthy fats like vegetable oils (extra-virgin olive, flaxseed, walnut, sesame) and vinegars (apple cider, white, red, balsamic, raspberry, rice) with herbs and spices, and a little salt and pepper.
- **Optional:** Whole grains (brown rice, quinoa, farro, whole-wheat pasta/bread) contain fiber and protein, and can round out your meal salad.

It's good to be aware of unhealthy salad ingredients (the ones that are often found in salad bars), which tend to be laden with a lot of saturated fats, salt, sugars, and refined carbs:

- Bacon bits or deli meats
- Mayonnaise-based salads (like potato, egg, and macaroni salad)
- Breaded and/or fried foods (breaded eggplant, fried tofu)
- Creamy dressing, most commercial dressings (these could be made with unhealthy oils or contain a lot of sugar, salt, and other chemicals)
- Croutons, sesame sticks, crispy chow mein noodles

Tips to Make the Habit Stick

- The healthiest salad is the one you make at home. Experiment with well-balanced meal salads until you have some go-to favorites.
- Try the Niçoise-Style Sardine Salad in Appendix A.

52. Make Your Own Healthy Meals at Home

Scientific studies have shown that people who cook their own food eat a wider variety of healthier food and tend to be a healthier weight. Takeout and delivery foods tend to be higher in refined carbs and saturated fats than home-cooked meals (think pizza, subs, or Chinese food). Home-cooked meals don't have to be complicated and can be very fast—even faster than the delivery person.

You can make quick home cooking easier in several steps. First, experiment with recipes when you have more time. This way you can learn what you like best and how to prepare it when you're not under pressure. Then pick your favorites that can be your go-tos for crazy evenings. Make sure the ingredients you'll need are always in stock in your kitchen or make extra and freeze for later. Then rotate your favorite meals regularly.

Tips to Make the Habit Stick

- When you have downtime, check out recipe ideas online. I love Pinterest for this reason. Type in "healthy dinners" and find hundreds of free recipes that you can pin to try later. Or subscribe to a healthy cooking magazine and bring it with you next time you go to the dentist or auto repair shop. I bet it'll be better reading than what's in the waiting room.

- Time your meal prep. You can use an inexpensive kitchen timer, stopwatch, or the timer on your phone. See how long it takes to put your recipe together. Pick ones that can be ready in 10–15 minutes, tops, and put them in your regular rotation.

- Stock up. Most quick meals will involve foods from your pantry and freezer that you can literally throw together. Make sure you have everything you need in doubles or triples.

- Prep ahead. If you're chopping an onion or peppers (or anything) for a recipe, but it doesn't call for the entire vegetable, chop the whole thing and store the extra in the fridge or freezer for use another day. It barely takes a minute while you're chopping anyway, and it saves you critical time later.
- Freeze for later. When you cook, make more than you need and freeze the extra. You can do this with ingredients that can be tossed into a recipe (whole grains like farro, quinoa, and brown rice freeze well) or with whole meals (soups and chilis especially).

53. Brown-Bag It

Many studies have shown that preparing food at home is associated with a healthier diet as well as a lower BMI. You can learn how to prepare meals to take to work or school. A study of more than forty thousand adults found that when people make their own lunch to bring to work and school, not only is their food intake healthier, but their weight also tends to be lower than in those who don't. It doesn't have to be anything fancy, and it should be something balanced and satisfying. Making your own meals for home and away can be key for losing weight and maintaining weight loss.

Tips to Make the Habit Stick

- When you make a healthy, balanced home-cooked meal, make extra so that you have leftovers. When you're cleaning up, package the extra in portable containers for weekday lunches. Make sure to pack a satisfying amount of food.
- You can also make lunches the night before and pack them up, so you just need to grab them on the way out the door. These can be as simple as veggies and dip with yogurt and fruit for dessert.

54. Be Restaurant Savvy

Of course you'll eat at restaurants or order takeout sometimes. Get in the habit of being restaurant savvy. There are several tactics that can help you stick to your healthy eating plan.

Tips to Make the Habit Stick

- Know your restaurant. If you're familiar with the offerings, you can decide ahead of time what you'll be eating. Even if it's a new place, nowadays you can quickly pull up the menu online and check out what it has. If you go in with a plan, you're less likely to order something that's not good for you.

- Remember to drink water. Thirst can be confused with hunger, and drinking water can help you eat less. Water with lemon or seltzer can be very refreshing and has no calories.

- Have a healthy salad first. Most restaurants have salads on the menu, and you can ask them to hold the toppings you don't need (bacon crumbles or croutons, for example) and to serve the dressing on the side.

- If the salads don't pique your interest, maybe a healthy appetizer does. Shrimp cocktail (with minimal dipping sauce, as it is typically loaded with sugar and salt), oysters on the half shell, and sashimi are high in protein as well as sources of heart-healthy omega-3 fats.

- Even if you order something really indulgent, you don't have to eat it all. Get in the habit of eating half your entrée and taking the other half home for another meal.

55. Be Prepared with Balanced Snacks

Sometimes you're stuck working late or caught in traffic or running a few errands that turned into half your day. It may have been a long time since your last healthy meal. Knowing this, it's key to have healthy and satisfying snacks on hand when you really need them.

Many snack foods are full of sugars and/or refined carbs (think candy bars, cookies, muffins, many granola bars, chips, pretzels, etc.). These will cause your blood sugar to spike up and then down, and you'll get shaky, dizzy, and cranky, and be hungry an hour after you eat.

A healthy snack is nice, but if it's too light, you'll be starving again in seconds. You want a filling, balanced snack, which will ideally have a little of everything that's good for you: healthy carbs (like complex carbohydrates and fiber), protein, fat, and nutrients.

Tips to Make the Habit Stick

- Balanced and satisfying snacks include things like ¼ cup or so of nuts or nut butter (and seeds or seed butter!) and a piece of fruit. Keep some at home and at work. Try to always be stocked up with fresh fruits that last a few days, like apples and oranges.
- A favorite late-afternoon pick-me-up of mine is two squares of dark chocolate and a creamy low-sugar, high-protein yogurt. That and a cup of tea will get me hours of productivity without tummy rumbling.

What Not to Eat: Foods to Avoid for Healthy Weight Loss

Everyone agrees that there are certain foods to avoid if you want to lose weight.

56. Run Away from Sugars and Refined Carbs

There are so many diets out there that it can seem overwhelming. Low-fat, low-carb, low-carb high-fat (LCHF), South Beach, Atkins, ketogenic, Weight Watchers, DASH, Whole30, and, of course, the Mediterranean diet. But if you look closer, you see that these diets have something in common: they all discourage sugars and refined grains and encourage vegetables. They differ in other ways, yes, but do the details matter?

A much-awaited, highly publicized head-to-head comparison study of the low-fat versus low-carb approaches found that either worked just as well for weight loss, provided that subjects avoided refined carbohydrates and added sugars, learned to better manage stress (i.e., not stress-eating), and exercised. The six hundred participants were split into two groups: low-fat and low-carb. They avoided sugary drinks (sodas, juices) and foods made with refined flours (like white bread and pastas, many breakfast cereals, cookies, and cake). The low-fat participants ate fruits and veggies; whole grains (like oats, brown rice, and quinoa); lentils and beans; fish, chicken; and low-fat dairy. The low-carb participants ate veggies, salmon, avocados, nuts and seeds (and butters made from them), hard cheeses, grass-fed meats, and plenty of olive oil. Participants in both groups were encouraged to make their own meals and eat sitting down at a table. Here's what's amazing: there were neither portion limits nor calorie-counting, yet participants in both groups lost an average of 12 pounds.

The bottom line is: if your goals include lasting weight loss and a healthy heart, you'll do best by avoiding added sugars and refined carbohydrates and eating more fruits and vegetables.

Tips to Make the Habit Stick

- Make certain areas of the grocery store "red zones." Learn where the sugars and refined carbs are in the grocery store and don't go there. The bakery section and the cereal and snack food aisles are examples of red zones.

- Build a better breakfast menu. Many common breakfast foods are chock-full of sugars and flours, like muffins, bagels, pancakes, waffles, and many cereals too. Move away from all of those and make healthier choices your go-to breakfast foods. Fruits, yogurt, nuts, oats, even eggs with vegetables are all far healthier. See the breakfast recipes at the end of the book!

The Natural Sugar in Fruit: Don't Worry about It

There are two measures of sugar in food: the glycemic index and the glycemic load. The glycemic index isn't very useful, because it neither takes into account portion sizes nor predicts the impact on our blood sugar levels. The glycemic load does. While the glycemic index of fruit is high, the glycemic load is low. The reason? Fruit eaten whole has a lot of water, healthy carbs, and fiber (and innumerable plant nutrients like vitamins, minerals, and antioxidants), all of which blunt the effect of natural fruit sugars in our body. So long as you don't remove all of that goodness by juicing, the overall effect of fruit is a healthy one.1 ounce of 100-proof spirits.

57. Search for Sneaky Added Sugars

You may be drinking more sugar than you realize. Juice can hide an unbelievable amount of sugar. Let's look at some labels: an 8-ounce glass of orange juice has 22 grams (6 teaspoons) of sugar, and that's even less than apple juice (28 grams = 7 teaspoons) or grape juice (36 grams = 9 teaspoons). Would you ever put 6, 7, or 9 teaspoons of sugar in anything you drink? Fancy bottled juices are no better, even if they throw in some healthy greens or protein. If you've been drinking juices or smoothies, look at the labels and see how many grams of sugar are in them. Four grams of sugar is equal to 1 teaspoon. There may be a lot in there, and as it's processed (blended), it's absorbed quickly in your body and causes insulin levels to spike. That causes the sugar to get stored as fat. Your best bet is to skip the juices and smoothies and drink water (or eat the fruit whole) instead.

Another sneaky sugar source is sauces and condiments. Bottled salad dressings can contain an unbelievable amount of sugar, as can ketchup, barbecue sauce, and sweet and sour sauce. Check the labels!

Tips to Make the Habit Stick

- Drink water, seltzer, unsweetened coffee, or tea. But don't drink sodas, sweetened beverages, or juice. Juicing is very in style right now, and there is nothing good about it.
- Miss juice? Squeeze some lemon or lime juice into your ice water. A squirt of lemon in your drink or food is fine.
- Be aware of added sugars in salad dressings and sauces. Learn how to make your own!

58. Avoid Artificial Sweeteners

Most studies of artificial sweeteners show that these are not associated with weight loss, but rather with weight gain. One possible explanation for this finding is that the sweetness triggers our brain to expect sugar, which causes a spike in insulin. That in turn pulls blood sugar into our fat cells, plumping them up. Basically, it's not only the calories in sugar that are bad for us; it's sweetness itself!

Over time, our taste buds adjust to a lower level of sweetness. People who cut out added sugars and artificial sweeteners often marvel at the natural sweetness of fruit. Remember, we aren't at all worried about the natural sugars in fruit, because fruit is a complete package including fiber and plant nutrients: sweetness as nature intended!

Tips to Make the Habit Stick

- Don't think you can adjust to no sweetener in your coffee, tea, or yogurt? Just use less.
- Try Mexican spiced coffee: a teaspoon of 100 percent pure cocoa, a sprinkle of cinnamon, and a splash of milk or cream of your choice.
- What about pancakes and French toast? Well, if you're going to enjoy these special treats, make them whole wheat and enjoy them with plenty of fruit, along with a modest pour of real, 100 percent natural honey, maple syrup, or agave syrup. It's better to ingest less-processed natural sweeteners than chemicals.

How to Eat: Eating Habits for Healthy Weight Loss

How we serve and consume our food can also impact weight.

59. Serve Buffet-Style, Not Family-Style

Leaving serving platters full of food right in the middle of the table encourages people to eat more. It's too easy to reach for seconds if the food is right there in front of you. But if you wait a bit, you'll give your body more time to get the "I'm full" signal. Here's a tip: When you cook a meal, leave the food in the kitchen and serve from there. The food will be out of sight and at a distance. Yes, people can go and get their seconds, but they have to get up to do it.

Tips to Make the Habit Stick

- Make it a new thing in your home that dinner is served buffet-style from the kitchen stove or counter. No platters or bowls of food on the table during meals.
- When the meal is over, put leftovers away. If they're left out, people will continue to pick.

60. Control Portion Size

It's well known that portions have become more and more supersized. Unfortunately, human stomachs can stretch, which has allowed us to eat bigger and bigger meals. Fortunately, our stomachs can also shrink.

Research studies show that when people use a large plate, they fill it with food and eat all of it. If they use a small plate, they still fill it with food and eat it but feel just as satisfied. Your eyes see a plate, but to your brain, it doesn't matter if it's a large one or a small one. So use a small plate.

If you've become accustomed to large meals, the idea of cutting back can be daunting. But if your meals are high in fiber (fruits, veggies, beans, lentils, whole grains) and include protein and healthy fats, you should feel full for a long time. Enjoying plenty of healthy fluid with your meal (water, seltzer, unsweetened tea) will help as well. This will make it easier to eat a smaller amount of food without feeling deprived or leaving the table hungry. You need to stick to this way of eating for life, so you need to feel good about it!

Tips to Make the Habit Stick

- Many patients of mine who have lost weight have done so using the "salad plate" tip: instead of using a full-sized dinner plate at meals, they use a smaller salad plate. They eat less but feel satisfied.
- Restaurants tend to serve extremely large portions, more than we need. As soon as you get your food, decide how much of it you're going to eat. Draw a line with your fork and literally push what you're not going to eat a little to the side. Then, ask the server to package it for you so you can enjoy it the next day. Two meals for the price of one!

61. Focus on Your Food

Distracted eating is associated with eating more of less healthy foods. Studies show that when we eat in front of the TV or computer, we take in a larger amount than when we eat at a table.

Mindful eating, on the other hand, is well associated with weight loss. Mindful eating means being present and aware during meals, paying attention to flavors and textures, savoring the food. It can help to get into the habit of eating slowly, chewing every mouthful thoroughly, and sipping water between bites. These mindfulness techniques help us enjoy what we're eating and eat less of it. Not only that, but there are important physiological effects: eating slowly means food ends up in the intestines slowly, where it's absorbed slowly. This means less of a blood sugar spike and likely better digestion. This also allows our brain to get the "I'm full" signal, which usually takes about 20 minutes. Waiting awhile before heading for seconds can have similar effects.

Traditionally meals were enjoyed over a couple of hours and among family and friends. Nowadays we tend to eat quickly, whether at home, on the road, or at our desk. Let's bring back some of that leisurely mealtime for our health.

Tips to Make the Habit Stick

- Make it a habit to sit down to eat, ideally always at a table.
- Do not allow phones, laptops, or other electronics at the table.
- Make it a rule: no eating in front of the TV (or computer or movies…).
- If you can, eat meals with others and chat.
- Drink water in between bites of food.

62. When You're Done, You're Done

Take action to signal the end of a meal. This helps prevent unnecessary second helpings or after-meal snacking. If you're legitimately still hungry, then you haven't had a full and balanced meal and may need to add fiber-full veggies, legumes, or whole grains to your plate. You should feel satisfied (but not uncomfortably full) after a meal. When you feel that you've had enough, develop a habit of "ending" your meal with a deliberate action (or two).

Tips to Make the Habit Stick

- When you've had enough to eat, place your napkin on your plate or even take your plate up to the sink.
- Pack up all the leftovers and put them away. If they're sitting out, people will pick.
- Brushing your teeth after eating is a wonderful strategy for not only your heart health but also your dental hygiene (remember Habit #48).
- Many people declare the kitchen "closed" after dinner and cleanup.

63. Limit Snacking by Distracting

Distract yourself from food cravings. Studies show that if you can do something else for 10 minutes, most cravings subside. Get up and do some stretches or take a walk. Or tell yourself that you'll do just one more quick task before you get that snack…usually the craving will pass.

Still hungry? Ask yourself if you're hungry enough to eat an apple. If you aren't, you're not really hungry. If you are, eat an apple.

Tips to Make the Habit Stick

- If you feel a craving for something not on your healthy list, take a quick walk around, even if it's only to the window or to another room. Changing your environment (even just the view or the furnishings) removes the craving cue, and often it disappears.
- Have something cold or hot. An icy beverage or hot tea can so occupy the taste and temperature receptors in your mouth that the craving melts away.
- Always have apples (or other produce) around for healthy snacking.

64. Don't Deprive Yourself, But Stay in Control

We've all been ambushed by well-intentioned friends, relatives, and coworkers who show up with the one food we cannot turn down. Sometimes, there's a really truly amazing treat that you just have to have. You know what? That's fine! You can enjoy the special foods you love and still maintain your healthy eating plan. As a matter of fact, you're more likely to stick to your eating plan if you don't deprive yourself. Here's how.

Decide what you're going to eat and then decide how much. Never eat right out of a bag or a bowl. Measure the portion and put it on a small plate before you start to eat. Make it last. Make it memorable. Then move on. (I call this the MMMM strategy: Measure, Make it last, Make it memorable, then Move on.)

(If you find that you cannot stop yourself and a taste of something triggers a binge, then see Chapter 8: Addressing Heart-Harmful Habits.)

Tips to Make the Habit Stick

- When you see something on your "unhealthy" list and your brain goes, "MMMM, I want that!" remember the MMMM strategy: Measure, Make it last, Make it memorable, then Move on.

- Mentally practice. This exercise is crucial: imagine what foods you can't turn down and then decide what your normal serving size would look like. How much would satisfy you? Picture yourself putting exactly the amount you decided on a small plate and then imagine enjoying every bite, chewing slowly. Think about how you may signal that you're done. Clear your plate, push it away, get up from the table, drink some water—whatever works for you.

- Physically practice your personal strategy. If what you imagined didn't work so well and you ended up indulging more than you planned, that's okay, and it's a great learning opportunity. You're creating your healthy eating plan for life, so there's no failing, only learning.

What to Do: Actions for Healthy Weight Loss

You probably already know that losing weight (and keeping it off) is about more than food.

65. Make It a Team Effort

Having a friend, partner, or group doing the same healthy plan really helps people stick with it and lose more weight. This is a large part of the reason that formal group-based lifestyle change programs really work. This may also be one of the reasons that many people have success after joining groups like Weight Watchers and Overeaters Anonymous. Being part of a "team" provides emotional support as well as accountability.

Tips to Make the Habit Stick

- You don't have to pay for a formal lifestyle change program or join a weight loss support group to benefit from the team approach. Maybe there's a friend or neighbor who wants to lose weight as well. If you promise a friend that you'll walk with her and then have a healthy breakfast in the mornings, you're more likely to follow through.
- Consider joining Weight Watchers, even if it's online. Online support groups can be just as effective as in-person support groups!
- Consider an office pool with a prize for the most weight lost. Everyone contributes a few dollars, and the winner gets the loot. My office has done this a few times, and everyone gets enthused and engaged! We've also committed to healthy snack and lunch options for most events, like antipasto platters or build-your-own-tacos with plenty of veggies.

66. Exercise!

Exercise is important for weight loss, maintenance of weight loss, stress management, and heart health. It's also very helpful for emotional eating, also called *stress eating*. In a 2013 survey of almost two thousand adults in the US, 38 percent reported overeating or eating unhealthy foods because they felt stress, and half reported doing so at least once a week. Research suggests that exercising can help curb stress as well as unhealthy stress eating. Of course exercise also burns calories and builds muscle, which boosts metabolism. There are multiple mechanisms through which regular exercise helps us lose extra weight. Chapter 7 is all about working exercise into your regular day.

Tips to Make the Habit Stick

- Get an inexpensive step counter or use the one on your smartphone. See how many steps there are in all the common things you do every day: the walk to your car in the morning, or around the block with the dog, or to the coffee machine at work… This can inspire you to get up and take little walks throughout the day, as a part of your regular everyday life.
- Aim for 10,000 steps a day, which is about 5 miles. No need for a treadmill or the gym.
- The next time you're forced to wait for a delayed flight or train or ride, consider it a blessing and an excuse to exercise. Don't sit on the nearest bench and pull out your phone. Walk around! Most people can get in about 500 steps over 15 minutes, and there are about 2,000 steps in a mile. So for every quarter-hour of delay, you can get in a quarter mile of walking. Bonus! You'll never feel inconvenienced again.

67. Monitor Your Intake

Multiple studies have shown that tracking your food intake is associated with weight loss. Logging food intake can be low-tech (like a little spiral-bound notebook with daily dietary choices scribbled in) or high-tech (like a smartphone fitness app). In a study of more than two thousand people participating in a diet and lifestyle program, logging food intake for even only three days a week was associated with clinically significant weight loss (5 percent of total body weight) at six months. For a 250-pound person, that's 12½ pounds! Scientists hypothesize that when we keep track of our intake, we become more aware of what we're eating, which helps us make healthier choices and consume less overall.

Tips to Make the Habit Stick

- Even if you're not yet ready to change your eating habits, it can be eye-opening to log your food and become aware of what you're consuming every day. Without changing your diet at all, log your daily food intake using a free app like MyFitnessPal, Lose It!, or SparkPeople.

- Apps can be intimidating, so a consultation with a nutritionist can help. A nutritionist (there are different kinds—see Chapter 2) can help you calculate what you eat on a typical day, as well as sort out what you should eat and how to keep track.

68. Weigh Yourself Regularly

Studies show that people who weigh themselves regularly are more likely to stick to a healthy weight loss plan and to successfully lose weight. In a study of two thousand people participating in a diet and lifestyle program, people who weighed in at least three days per week lost at least 5 percent of their total body weight after six months.

People who have a history of an eating disorder, however, should be careful about systematically weighing themselves, as this action can be triggering and is not medically advised. For people who do not have that history and sincerely want to drop some pounds, the experts advise that you are less likely to lose weight if you are not following your weight, so get a scale.

Tips to Make the Habit Stick

- If you don't have a scale at home, consider getting a simple one. No need to get a smart scale that syncs to your phone and watch.
- Weigh yourself at about the same time of day, and without clothes, for more consistent comparisons.

69. Stick to a Routine

People who have a regular routine (eating basically the same things and doing the same activities at roughly the same times) are more successful with losing weight and maintaining a healthy weight. That's because the more you stick to a routine, the more automatic it becomes, and the stronger the habit grows. If you find healthy meals and activities that you particularly enjoy and that work for your life, then stick to those choices. You'll be more likely to revert to those same healthy choices, even in times of turmoil, travel, or stress. It will become habit.

Tips to Make the Habit Stick

- Try different recipes and see what you like. Rotate a few meal options until you see weight coming off. Keeping things the same and stable makes it a lot easier to stick to your plan.
- Try to eat at roughly the same times every day. This will make you less likely to mindlessly eat something unhealthy that's put in front of you at an odd time, like the box of baked goods that someone just brought to your office.
- If you're working stress management and physical activity into your life, try to choose a few practices you can build into your daily schedule. Repeat, repeat, repeat.

70. Reward Yourself for All of Your Achievements

If you're keeping track of your physical activity, healthy eating, stress management strategies, and weight loss, you can reward yourself for your progress. This is a very effective strategy for establishing new habits. Here's the thing: you want to pick very small achievements and very healthy rewards. This is so that you can set yourself up for success, which helps the habit take hold.

With weight loss, it's especially important to stick to small, specific, measurable achievements, and weight is only one of them. If you're monitoring your food intake, reward yourself for every three days of logging. If you have a step counter, you can reward yourself for meeting your step goal for three days in a row. Get the idea? If you're able to keep track, you can pat yourself on the back.

However, choosing unhealthful treats as a reward would undermine your efforts and disrupt your success. So chocolate bars are not a good reward (unless it's the two small squares of dark chocolate that's so good for your heart that I recommended in Chapter 5). The best rewards will help you achieve even more: new cooking equipment, workout gear, fitness gadgets, yoga classes, massage treatments… And they don't have to be big or expensive things. Cooking equipment rewards can be small, like a new citrus squeezer, a steamer basket, a silicone barbecue brush, oven mitts; or big, like a set of good kitchen knives. Workout gear could mean anything from new socks to a wicking T-shirt to thermal running pants. Fitness gadgets range from $10 step counters to $300 smart watches. Yoga classes can be $10 each or require a membership. A massage could be a freebie from your partner or a professional sports massage from a trainer. There's a huge range of possibilities here. The idea is to keep track of your efforts and progress so that you can reward yourself for a job well done.

Tips to Make the Habit Stick

- Pick some very small and easily attainable goals. Examples include logging your food, meeting your daily steps goal, or meditating for three days in a row. How about servings of fruits and vegetables? For every three days you eat at least 4 to 5 cups of fruits and vegetables, you get a reward. Or every three days you bring your own lunch to work. Three days too little? Nothing is too little! Every effort counts, and you want to set yourself up for success early on.
- Pick some healthy rewards and write down what you'll get when you achieve each small goal. Then follow through!

Troubleshooting Habits for Healthy Weight Loss

Eating a plant-based diet plus avoiding added sugars and refined grains can result in very significant weight loss for many people, but it doesn't work for everyone right away. Have you given it long enough? If it's only been a week or two, think about giving it more time.

But maybe you've given it time, and it's not working. I know you can lose weight; we just haven't figured out what works for you yet. So let's figure it out. This means reevaluating and adjusting what you're eating, how you're eating, what you're doing, and, most importantly, how you're feeling.

What You're Eating

First check to make sure you're eating a healthy plant-based diet and avoiding unhealthy added sugars and refined grains. If you are, then here are some more suggestions.

71. Consider Limiting Flours and Starches

Many people experience significant weight loss using a low-carbohydrate diet (like the Paleo, LCHF, and ketogenic diets). These diets include mostly vegetables, plus high-protein fish, eggs, all kinds of meats, a lot of fatty nuts, nut butter, and avocados, with very little fruits and no legumes or grains. While this works well for weight loss, it's difficult to stick to forever. (No fruits? No legumes or whole grains? Those are superhealthy foods!) Also, there's not a lot of evidence to suggest that this approach is heart-healthy. After all, it's missing all the plant nutrients and fiber in fruits, legumes, and whole grains.

But we can combine the weight loss benefits of a low-carbohydrate approach with the heart-healthy benefits of a plant-based diet by simply limiting flours and starches. There's no need to switch diets or completely eliminate foods; we can just eat more of some foods and less of others.

Tips to Make the Habit Stick

- Eat more of:
  - Colorful and cruciferous vegetables (broccoli, cauliflower, cabbage, Brussels sprouts, bell peppers, carrots)
  - Greens (spinach, kale, chard, collards)
  - High-fiber fruits like berries (blueberries, strawberries, raspberries); apples; oranges; pears
  - Healthy fats (avocados, nuts, seeds, vegetable oils)
- Eat some of:
  - Proteins (legumes like beans, lentils, peas, and tofu, and fish and chicken)
  - Intact whole grains (quinoa, oats, brown rice, farro)
  - Colorful starchy vegetables (sweet potatoes, squash)

(Note: studies show that colorful starchy veggies and legumes are healthy and compatible with weight loss.)

- Eat less of:
  - Starchy white vegetables (white potatoes)
  - Starchy white fruits (bananas)
  - Processed grains of all kinds (foods made with flours, such as cereals, pastas, breads [even ones made with whole-grain flours])

This will give you a lower-carb, plant-based diet that still has all the heart-healthy benefits you need.

Check Your Meal Makeup

Make sure you're eating mostly plants, like actual fruits and vegetables. "Vegetarian" and "vegan" diets can easily consist of something other than plants. Just ask my friend who gained a substantial amount of weight while experimenting with veganism: she ate cereals, breads, and pastas at every meal. Cereals, breads, and pastas, even ones made from whole grains, are high in carbohydrates. Plant-based means plants, so make sure about half of your daily intake is fruits and vegetables.

72. Is Alcohol Undermining Your Efforts?

One glass of red or white wine, one beer, or one mixed drink (not made with juice) a day may be good for your heart, but is it enabling unhealthy snacking? Alcohol is famous for lowering our inhibitions, and this often means eating things we wouldn't eat otherwise. Not many people have a beer and then say, "Hey, pass that salad; it looks really good." More often it's, "Hey, pass the wings; they look really good."

Not only that, but alcoholic beverages have calories too. They're not particularly nutrition calories either.

Tips to Make the Habit Stick

- Enjoy wine with dinner? Always have a glass of water or seltzer first, as well as between every glass of wine.
- Know you tend to order the unhealthy apps when you have a beer? Order something healthy to enjoy first so you're a little full when the wings hit the table.
- Having trouble limiting to one drink? You may want to abstain completely while trying to lose weight.
- If you are unable to abstain, this could be due to self-medicating with alcohol, or alcohol use disorder, so please seek the advice of a healthcare provider. (This is covered more extensively in Chapter 8: Addressing Heart-Harmful Habits, under "Alcohol Use Disorder.")

73. Consider a More Individualized Plan

A scientific review of numerous diets found that all were equal in terms of weight loss. The author concluded: "Weight loss occurs with many different diets and there are no clear conclusions on the optimal diet, apart from the diet which the individual can stick to long-term, whatever the composition." So, generally speaking, just about any diet can help people lose weight, if they can stick to it...but "people" is not *you*. Your plan may need to be individualized. In many cases, consulting with a nutrition expert can be extremely helpful. In Chapter 2, we reviewed the different types of nutrition experts. You may want to seek out a registered dietitian who has the credentials that reflect a certain standard of training.

Tips to Make the Habit Stick

- Check to see if your insurance covers a nutritionist consult, and then ask your doctor for a referral to the appropriate expert.
- Many gyms offer inexpensive nutrition consults; check yours out.

How You're Eating

How we eat, specifically the timing of our meals, can greatly impact weight loss or gain for some people.

74. Consider Intermittent Fasting

You can also adjust the timing of your eating to promote weight loss. In intermittent fasting, people go some period without eating, only drinking water, tea, coffee, or broth. It works, and here's why: when we eat, food digested in our intestines gets broken down into sugars, which end up in our bloodstream. While our cells use some of that for energy, insulin makes sure that any extra gets stored as fat. Insulin is a hormone made in the pancreas and is secreted when we eat. The more we eat, and especially the more processed carbohydrates we eat, the more insulin is secreted. Insulin brings sugar into the fat cells and keeps it there. But between meals (as long as we don't snack), our insulin levels will go down, and the sugar stored in our fat cells can be released and used as energy. Intermittent fasting allows our insulin levels to go down, so we use up our fat stores and lose weight.

New studies suggest that simply extending the overnight fast works as well as other forms of intermittent fasting and can be far more manageable. This makes a lot of sense, because we have evolved to be in sync with the night/day cycle (i.e., circadian rhythm). We're supposed to eat in the daytime and sleep in the nighttime. Nighttime eating is well associated with a higher risk of obesity, as well as diabetes. In one study, obese men with prediabetes tried two approaches: an extended overnight fast (only eating between seven a.m. and three p.m.) or eating throughout the whole day. After five weeks, the extended overnight fast group had significantly lower insulin levels and improved insulin sensitivity, as well as ten-point improvements in systolic and diastolic blood pressures. Studies like this and others suggest that when a healthy diet and exercise aren't working, extending your usual overnight fast could really help you lose weight. This approach is even recommended by specialists working with patients who already have diabetes. Metabolic expert Deborah Wexler, MD, Director of the Massachusetts General Hospital Diabetes Center and associate professor at Harvard Medical School, states: "There is evidence to suggest that the circadian rhythm fasting approach, where meals are restricted to an 8- to 10-hour period of the daytime, is effective." She counsels her patients who would benefit from weight loss about this approach.

Tips to Make the Habit Stick

- Follow the basic plant-based diet outlined in this book: eat fruits, vegetables, legumes, whole grains, lean proteins, and healthy fats, and avoid sugars and refined grains.
- Extend your overnight fast. Take all your food in an 8-hour period of the day, and, for best effect, make it earlier in the day. This can be seven a.m. to three p.m., ten a.m. to six p.m., or even twelve p.m. to eight p.m. Just make sure you're done eating by nightfall and then fast for 16 hours.
- Even if your 8-hour period is later, don't eat a meal just before bed-time. Try to consistently avoid any snacking or eating at nighttime.

What You're Doing

Consider some additional actions that can greatly impact weight.

75. Build Muscle, Boost Metabolism

Many people need more than cardio to help them lose weight and keep it off. Muscle-building exercises like weight lifting, working out with kettle-bells, resistance training with machines, or Pilates can get those numbers on the scale down. This is especially true for people with or at risk for diabetes, older individuals, and peri- and post-menopausal women. Remember, when we eat, insulin brings any extra sugar that is not used as fuel into the fat cells, making us fatter. What we want is for any extra sugar to get used up as fuel for our muscles and not be stored as fat. When we burn fat for fuel, we lose weight. A lower-carb, plant-based diet and/or intermittent fasting are both safe and natural lifestyle approaches that help keep blood sugars low and force our body to use fat for fuel. But we can boost those approaches by building more muscle and then working it. More muscle will need more fuel and working it will burn more fuel. Muscle is lean body mass, and it's really good for us.

Tips to Make the Habit Stick

- You don't have to lift weights to build muscle. Your core muscles are large muscle groups deep in your torso and pelvis, and there are many safe and easy exercises to help you build them up. Many of these can be done on a mat on the floor. Try taking a Pilates class, either at a gym, on DVD or cable, or online.
- If you don't know where to start, a trainer can help.

76. Fortify Your Foundation

Remember back in Chapter 4, we learned how important stress management and sleep are. Stress and insufficient sleep trigger the release of hormones like cortisol, which is bad for your heart and circulation. Cortisol also contributes to fat storage, causing more fat to be formed and blocking fat from being used as energy. Both chronic stress and insufficient sleep are well associated with weight gain and obesity. If you're having trouble losing weight, consider: are you feeling stressed out? Are you getting enough good sleep?

Tips to Make the Habit Stick

- Is stress causing you to overeat? Stress eating can be managed with awareness and good stress management techniques. However, there are different forms of overeating, and we will address these in more detail in Chapter 8.
- Practice self-care and stress management techniques every day. If yoga is effective for you, try to do a few poses every morning or evening. If you enjoy walking, schedule a walk into your day every day.
- If you're struggling to work stress management techniques into your life, talk to a mental health professional, like a therapist. She can help you figure this out.
- If you're not sleeping enough, or if your sleep is poor, it can be helpful to speak to a healthcare provider to see if this is due to an underlying medical sleep disorder (like sleep apnea) or something else, like insomnia. Remember from Chapter 4 that the best treatments for insomnia are behavioral and can include working toward a consistent sleep/wake schedule and bedtime routine, as well as specialized cognitive behavioral therapy. Additional testing, medications, therapy, or a continuous positive airway pressure machine (CPAP, a treatment for sleep apnea) may also be prescribed.

77. Consider Consulting an Obesity Specialist

Research shows that when diet and lifestyle alone aren't working for weight loss, a specialist can help. Obesity medicine specialist Fatima Cody Stanford, MD, MPH, MPA, is an expert in the three main treatment approaches to obesity: diet and lifestyle, medications, and surgery. She always encourages a diet and lifestyle change program first but acknowledges that sometimes it's not enough. She emphasizes (and research supports) how helpful weight loss medications can be. "I listen to the patient," she said. "If they tell me that sugar is a trigger for them, then I believe them, because sugar can trigger appetite. If that's their trigger, then I think about what tool I can use to help them with their struggle. Medications affect the way the brain manages the body's weight set point and how the brain interacts with the environment." Research shows that weight loss medications aren't prescribed often enough, despite the fact that they can be useful for people.

Another option is weight loss surgery, and there are generally two options: gastric sleeve and gastric bypass. The gastric sleeve sews off part of the stomach, which decreases food intake and increases the feeling of fullness. Gastric bypass reroutes the intestines so that food enters a very small stomach pouch and bypasses the rest of the stomach and first part of the intestines. This decreases food intake, increases the feeling of fullness, and causes poor absorption of what does pass through the digestive tract. Both usually result in long-term weight loss—the gastric bypass procedure more so—with about 50 percent of excess weight still lost after ten years. To be eligible for these procedures, people must have a BMI over 40, or a BMI over 35 plus obesity-related disease such as obstructive sleep apnea, type 2 diabetes, severe high blood pressure, or heart disease.

Tips to Make the Habit Stick

- Primary care providers can prescribe weight loss medications, so if you feel that your diet and lifestyle efforts need a boost, talk to your doctor or ask for a referral to a reputable weight loss center. A list of certified obesity medicine specialists is available at www.abom.org.
- If you do find weight loss medications helpful, remember that they need to be taken long-term or weight can be regained.

You now have a good number of weight loss tools and suggestions that you can begin to incorporate into your life as habits. Let's move on to heart-healthy activity.

Chapter 7

Run (Walk, Dance, Garden...) for Your Life: Activity Habits

INACTIVITY IS TOXIC to your system, promoting inflammation and damage to your blood vessels and organs. However, if you give yourself good nutrition and physical activity every day, your body can heal, and you can live a good, long life.

When we move, we exercise our heart and flex our arteries, which boost our circulation and flush damaging inflammatory toxins away. There are still parts of the world where heart disease barely exists and people enjoy long and vibrant lives. They're not working out at a gym or running long-distance. They're walking, gardening, goat-herding, hiking…basic, easy, low-intensity activities that have huge benefits, when you do them every day. Studies show that regular physical activity improves blood pressure, lowers blood sugars and cholesterol, promotes weight loss, relieves stress, boosts mood, and is associated with lower risk for heart disease.

The Most Important Activity Habits for a Healthy Heart

Moving your body is critical for heart health, and all movement counts. Read this chapter and learn how you can make exercise a daily habit.

78. Redefine Exercise

All activity counts. You may already be getting in activity that you don't even realize. We often measure physical activity in metabolic equivalents (METS), where 1 MET is just sitting doing nothing, 2 METS is light activity, 3–6 METS is moderate activity, and more than 6 METS is vigorous activity. Here's a table of common activities and how many METS of physical activity they're worth:

Rest: 1 MET	Light Activity: 2 METS	Moderate Activity: 3–6 METS	Vigorous Activity: >6 METS
Sitting quietly	Sitting actively (fishing, playing an instrument); Standing (cooking, washing dishes)	Walking briskly (4 MPH); Housework (mopping, vacuuming, washing windows); Light yard work (walking power mower)	Jogging (6 MPH); Shoveling; Carrying heavy loads; Sports (basketball game, soccer game)

Source: Harvard T.H. Chan School of Public Health, The Nutrition Source, Measuring Physical Activity: www.hsph.harvard.edu/nutritionsource/mets-activity-table/

All activity counts, and it doesn't need to be at a gym. Even better if it's not, as that makes it easier to incorporate into your everyday life. Think of ways you're already active throughout the day. Congratulations! Think of how you can push for a little more daily activity. Take every opportunity to move your body throughout your regular day, because it all adds up!

Tips to Make the Habit Stick

- Are there stairs to get into your apartment or home? Are there stairs within your apartment or home? Think of how many flights you go up and down in a day. Can you work in a few more?
- Do you walk to get to your car, the train, or the bus? Walk briskly! Any way to add more steps? Maybe park farther away from home or walk around the block, just for fun.
- Do you ever need to take out the trash? Take as few items as possible out at a time so you get to walk back and forth more. Or take a walk around the block after the barrels are out.

79. Run for Your Life (for 5 Minutes a Day)

It does not take a lot of activity to provide benefits. In a 2014 analysis of fifteen years' worth of data from more than fifty-five thousand people, running for as little as 5–10 minutes a day was associated with a 45 percent reduced risk of death from heart attacks and strokes, as well as a 30 percent reduced risk of death from any cause. This benefit was seen even after accounting for age, sex, and weight, and correcting for other health risk variables such as high blood pressure, diabetes, smoking, and alcohol consumption. If you enjoy running at all, any running at all is excellent for your health.

Tips to Make the Habit Stick

- Get your workout gear ready the night before so you have no excuses in the morning.
- When you're feeling unmotivated, it's okay to tell yourself, "I'm only going to run for 5 minutes," and then only run for that long, because you'll still be doing yourself some good.
- Get bored while running? This can be an excellent time to listen to a good podcast or new music.

80. Inconvenience Yourself

Inconvenience conveniently becomes exercise! Any way you can rig your environment to encourage less sitting and more moving is a healthy move. There are a million ways you can inconvenience yourself, which will help you (force you, actually) to move around more.

Tips to Make the Habit Stick

- Park farther away from the store so you can get in more steps.
- Hide the TV remote so you have to manually change the channel or just put it at a distance so you have to get up to use it.
- If you're just picking up a few things from the grocery store, use a carry basket instead of a wheeled cart. Biceps curls while you shop!
- My personal favorite way to inconvenience myself is to always take the stairs, even up to the twenty-second floor of our hospital. For people who are physically able to climb stairs, this can be a bonus workout in the midst of any workday or errand. Leave the elevators and escalators free for those who really need them.

81. Stand Up for Yourself

They say sitting is the new smoking, and they're right. Prolonged sitting is associated with an increased risk of death, and the longer you sit, the higher the risk. One analysis looking at data from more than five hundred thousand people found that sitting for 10 or more hours per day was associated with a 34 percent higher risk of death—from any cause. Scientists think that when we sit, toxins also sit, which promotes damage to our blood vessels. This increases our risk for heart disease and related diseases (like peripheral arterial disease and strokes). But you have the power to lower your risk: another study showed that getting up and walking around once every hour reduced the damaging effect to blood vessels. So if there are times when you find yourself sitting for a while, stand up and move around.

Tips to Make the Habit Stick

- If your job requires a lot of sitting at a desk, stand up every 15 minutes to stretch and walk around at least every hour.
- Even better: get a standing desk. These do not need to be fancy and can even be jury-rigged using things like crates or piles of books. (My standing desk at home is a pile of textbooks stacked on our dining room buffet. I kid you not.)
- Watch a lot of TV? Stand up and stretch at every commercial break.
- Commute to work on a train? Try standing instead of sitting.

82. Housework Is Heart-Healthy

Yes, the work you do in and around the house counts as activity. In a 2017 study published in *The Lancet*, scientists looked at the effect of various activities on heart and related disease risk. They followed one hundred and thirty thousand participants from all over the world, including both low- and high-income countries and people of all races, for seven years. They found that it didn't matter if activity was recreational (fitness and sports) or non-recreational (related to work, domestic chores, or transportation); it was all beneficial. One hundred and fifty minutes per week of moderate physical activity was associated with a 20 percent reduction in risk for heart and related diseases, as well as a 28 percent reduction in risk of death from any cause. Remember Habit #78? Housework such as mopping and vacuuming is considered moderate physical activity. If you houseclean for 150 minutes per week (about 21 minutes a day), you're doing your body a lot of good.

Tips to Make the Habit Stick

- Look forward to your housework as a free workout with big heart benefits (with a bonus of clean floors).
- Think of other forms of housework that can count as moderate (or even vigorous) physical activity. Washing windows, decluttering rooms, carrying laundry baskets up and down stairs, reorganizing the garage...these count!
- Tally up your minutes of housework each day and week. Are you getting more than 21 minutes a day and 150 minutes per week? If so, congratulations. If not, add a few more minutes of housework here and there for added benefits (for your body and your living space).

83. Track Your Activity

Activity monitors can motivate you to move more. In an analysis of data from more than one thousand participants who were overweight and obese, wearing an activity monitor as part of a lifestyle change intervention was associated with significantly increased physical activity. In another research study of more than two thousand people participating in a diet and lifestyle program over six months, those who averaged 6,500 steps daily lost at least 5 percent of their total body weight, while those who averaged 8,000 steps lost at least 10 percent of their body weight. Keeping track of the number of steps helped participants reach higher goals.

An activity monitor can be anything from an inexpensive plastic step counter or a fancy fitness watch. You also can use a free app on your smartphone. Most smartphones come with a free health application that tracks steps per day, but there are many other free apps available, such as Pacer, Runkeeper, SparkPeople, and MyFitnessPal.

Tips to Make the Habit Stick

- Set a personal goal for steps walked per day. It's popular to aim for 10,000 steps per day (roughly 5 miles), but this is not based on any official guideline. Anything that's more than what you're already doing is fine.
- Find fun ways to add more steps per day. For me to walk to the office kitchen and back is exactly 100 steps, so every time I refill my water bottle I know I'm getting those steps in.
- Consider tracking flights of stairs climbed per day as well. This is considered a vigorous activity, similar to hiking or climbing mountains.

84. Exercise with Others

Group activities are fun. Signing up for a class or making a plan to meet up with people to exercise is motivating and helps us stick to a plan. These are also good ways to try out new activities.

Beyond all those pluses, there is a bigger one: exercising with others provides a sense of social connectedness, which has powerful mental health benefits. Remember from Chapters 1 and 2 that isolation and loneliness are associated with stress and depression, as well as with heart disease. Studies show that people who exercise alone or with others enjoy similar physical health benefits, but the more people exercise with others, the healthier they feel in body and in mind. The social aspect of group activity is heart-healthy, in every sense.

Tips to Make the Habit Stick

- Do you know anyone (whose company you enjoy) who also wants to live healthier? See if he'd like to walk, go to a gym, or take a yoga class with you.
- Find out if there are any fitness classes in your area. Many gyms offer a free one-day pass to interested individuals; yoga studios often offer a free one-class pass. Try out different types of activities and classes. People often become friends through these venues.
- Check out apps like SparkPeople, which has a "Buddy Finder" feature at www.sparkpeople.com/mypage_home.asp, or online group websites like *Meetup*. A 10-second search in my zip code results in hundreds of upcoming open fitness Meetups, including badminton, Ping-Pong, Frisbee, and "People That Can't Run Good." You can search through endless options to find an activity Meetup near you: www.meetup.com/.

85. Work Activity Into Your Workday

"I don't have time to exercise because I work a long day." You may work a long day, but you have time to exercise. You may already be getting more exercise than you realize: when my patient, an emergency room nurse, got a step counter, she realized that she logged well over her goal of 10,000 steps during her 10-hour emergency room shift. That was twice as many steps as she got when she went to the gym and walked on the treadmill. Your heart and blood vessels do not care if you're at the gym or at work. Feeling self-conscious? It's hip to be active. You commonly see people in business attire and sneakers these days. Standing desks and walking meetings are a thing. By getting up and moving around, you may inspire the people around you.

Tips to Make the Habit Stick

- Walk a few laps around your office when you go to the bathroom or get a coffee.
- Always take the stairs.
- Instead of sending an email, get up and go to a colleague's desk.
- No need to book a conference room: schedule a "walking meeting," where a topic is discussed while strolling rather than sitting.
- Does your job involve a lot of sitting at a computer? I strongly advise a standing desk. It doesn't have to be expensive or fancy. Standing is good for your core muscles and does wonders for chronic low back pain.

86. Exercise First Thing

So many things can get in the way of your plan to exercise in the afternoon. Working late, social events, kids' activities, neighborhood gatherings... If you're going to get in a workout, it's best to get it in early. This can be a 5-minute routine or an hour-long gym visit. Whatever it is, get it out of the way.

Tips to Make the Habit Stick

- Lay out your workout gear the night before, right in the area where you'll be getting dressed.
- Better yet, consider sleeping in your workout clothes.
- Make a commitment to someone else. Sign up for an early morning class at the gym, arrange to meet a neighbor for a walk, or just let your family know your intentions. You'll be more likely to get up in the morning.
- If you use a gym, and it's on the way to work, consider packing your work clothes so you can get a quick workout and shower there.

87. An Hour a Day Keeps the Grim Reaper Away...

We know that sitting for long periods during the day is associated with an increased risk of death from any cause. While this is true, all is not lost for people who have no other options. Maybe someone has a job that requires long hours of sitting, like sewing or driving a truck or a taxi. Regardless, just an hour a day of moderate physical activity can cancel out the increased risk of death from 8 hours a day of sitting. Researchers analyzed data from sixteen large studies including more than a million participants and found that 60–75 minutes per day of activities such as brisk walking; riding a bicycle; or playing golf, softball, or tennis eliminated the risk associated with sitting for 8 hours a day. Less time was required for more vigorous activities such as running, competitive cycling or Spinning, playing soccer, or singles tennis.

Even if your work requires long hours of sitting, reduce your risk of heart disease with an hour of moderate activity every day. This can be broken up into 10 minutes here and 10 minutes there throughout the day. It all counts!

Tips to Make the Habit Stick

- Got a dog? Walk the dog. This is good for your mental health as well (and the dog).
- When you are at work, find reasons to be active. Walk to the mailbox, to lunch, to get coffee. Take the stairs, and maybe some extra stairs!
- Do some jumping jacks first thing in the morning or try other easy, in-place calisthenics.
- If you have to wait for a train or plane, stand up and walk around.

88. Don't Sit in Front of the TV

TV sitting time is associated with even greater risk of death. Remember the study just discussed that showed how activity can cancel out the risk of death from prolonged sitting? Even more than an hour per day of moderate activity does not eliminate the risks associated with 5 or more hours per day of zoning in front of the tube.

Why the extra negative effect of TV watching? People are less likely to get up and walk around while watching TV than they are at work. In addition, people tend to watch TV in the evening after eating dinner, which may have negative effects on their blood sugar and fat metabolism. Or perhaps people are prompted to snack on unhealthy foods during those commercial breaks.

Tips to Make the Habit Stick

- If you love your TV, set a stationary bike squarely in front of it and attach the remote to the handlebars.
- Make it a rule that you're not allowed to watch TV while sitting on the couch. Become a person who does not watch TV while sitting on the couch.
- Consider watching your shows only at the gym on an iPad. Many gyms feature cardio equipment with personal screens for watching a wide variety of shows.

89. Multitask Your Workout

Is "I have too much work to do" often an excuse not to exercise? Or do you find that you get bored during workouts? Make your workouts count in other ways. Multitasking makes the time go faster as well!

Tips to Make the Habit Stick

- You can easily work on a tablet computer, iPad, or phone while exercising on a StairMaster, stair treadmill, or stationary bike. As a working mom, I can attest to this: I study, write, and shop while on the stair treadmill at the gym. A word of caution: make sure that you are able to keep your balance on the machine while you are looking at a screen. This may require keeping the workout intensity low to moderate.

- Do you enjoy watching TV? Watching your shows while exercising is fine (and will help you avoid the increased risk of death from sitting and watching TV).

- Need to catch up with an old friend, or is your mother expecting your call? Walk and talk!

90. Exercise Last Thing

Going to bed with food in your belly is a surefire way to gain weight. Besides not eating anytime close to bedtime, consider taking a stroll or other light exercise after dinner. This helps you use up some of the calories you just took in and promotes digestion. Make it a habit to do some gentle stretching and core exercises before bedtime. Even a 2- to 5-minute routine provides benefits if done regularly. This helps you unplug, stretches and relaxes your muscles, and builds core strength gently over time.

Tips to Make the Habit Stick

- Get your family, partner, or dog into the habit of an after-dinner stroll or other activity.
- After dinner and cleanup is a great time to do some housework, like switching laundry or picking up a room. That's activity and can help you achieve two goals at the same time (three if your after-dinner activity replaces sitting and watching TV!).

In summary, you've learned that when it comes to heart health, all physical activity counts, and the more the better. You now have numerous options for adding activity to your regular day, every day, and making activity a regular habit. If one of these habit suggestions doesn't work for you, try a different one. There are many ways to fit fitness into your life.

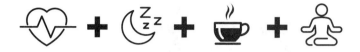

Chapter 8

Addressing Heart-Harmful Habits

THERE IS CLEARLY overlap between habit and addiction, and sometimes what we label as a bad habit is actually addiction. In this chapter you'll learn about the similarities and differences between habit and addiction, and how to recognize certain addictions. You'll learn approaches, techniques, and resources to effectively address common heart-harmful habits and addictions, like tobacco, alcohol, overeating, and electronics, and what steps to take if these aren't enough. Sometimes, addressing underlying mental health issues is the key to lasting lifestyle change.

Habit and Addiction Overview

Habits and addictions sometimes overlap. Let's look at what's similar and what's different between these two concepts.

Habit is defined as a something that you do over and over again so often that it becomes automatic. As we learned in Chapter 3, habits can involve brain pathways of craving and reward.

Addiction is defined as something that is so powerfully rewarding that you're compelled to keep doing it, despite negative consequences. This broad definition can be applied to a wide range of substances and behaviors, including tobacco; alcohol; overeating; gambling; and excessive Internet, phone, video game, or TV use.

While a habit can evolve into addiction, there are differences, and it's all about neurochemistry. In addiction, the brain pathways of craving and reward are very strongly involved, and the person can become physiologically dependent, experiencing withdrawal without the substance. For this reason, in medical and psychiatric diagnostic guidelines, addiction usually refers to substances like alcohol and drugs (including tobacco) and is called *substance use disorder*. But substances and behaviors can involve the same brain pathways, feature similar patterns, and sometimes respond to similar treatments, so we do recognize certain compulsive behaviors as a form of addiction, such as gambling disorder.

There are many substance and behavior habits that can become addictions. This chapter will focus on those that are most directly heart-unhealthy, including tobacco, alcohol, overeating, and electronics addiction.

Tobacco Use Disorder

One hundred years of data and experience show us just how dangerous smoking is for people. Smokers die an average of ten years earlier than nonsmokers and suffer from significantly more disease and disability. Thirty-two percent of all coronary heart disease deaths and 33 percent of all cancer deaths in the US are directly due to smoking. The tobacco industry was well aware of the health risks related to smoking but intentionally misled the public, all in the name of profits. As a matter of fact, today's high-tech cigarettes are worse for you than the originals: ventilated filters increase the flow of smoke to the lungs, allowing more toxins to be delivered deeper into the lung tissue. This is part of the reason smokers today are more likely to get lung cancer than smokers fifty years ago.

It's never too late to quit smoking. After a diagnosis of lung cancer, continuing to smoke makes cancer therapy less effective. Quitting smoking can boost treatment. Heart-health benefits can be seen in as little as an hour after quitting, as your heart rate and blood pressure begin to go down. After a number of months, arteries will be less stiff and blood pressures will be more normal; after a number of years, the risk of heart disease is significantly lower (compared to people who didn't quit).

The Most Important Habits for Quitting Smoking

If you smoke and you're interested in quitting, here are some suggestions.

91. A Plan Is More Important Than Motivation

Having a good quit plan in place before stubbing out that last ciga-rette is strongly associated with successful quitting. Tobacco is strongly addictive, and motivation alone is less likely to be effective against any addiction. In a good quit plan, you will want to understand your habit loop, anticipate challenges, and plan ahead. These tips are loosely based on the Centers for Disease Control and Prevention's Tips from Former Smokers at www.cdc.gov/tobacco/campaign/tips/quit-smoking/guide/ quit-plan.html.

Tips to Make the Habit Stick

- Understand why you want to quit. What's your main motivation? Write it down and put it where you can see it.
- Understand your smoking habit. What are your triggers? Think about all the things, places, and people that make you want to light up. Now for each, think about how you'll avoid or manage them. This is anticipating your challenges. Write them all down and keep that list handy, because you'll need it.
- Set a quit date. Make it far enough ahead that you can get your plan in place.
- Tell your family and friends that you plan to quit and when. Having their support can help you be successful.
- As you near your date, throw away or destroy all cigarettes and smoking-related paraphernalia. Do not keep "just one" hidden away "just in case," because you will smoke it.
- Remember that good stress management will help you quit. Consider going back and reading Chapter 4 so you have your stress management plan down.

92. Tie Your Quit Date to Another Event

Are you planning on taking a vacation, moving, or switching jobs? It can be very helpful to set your quit date at the same time. The change in surroundings disrupts the habit loop by removing your usual environmental triggers.

Tips to Make the Habit Stick

- Taking advantage of your upcoming change in environment by planning to quit smoking at the same time can really boost your quitting efforts. You still need to plan, though. Look at Habit #91 and make a good plan.
- Even if you aren't going anywhere, you can still use this technique. Is there another event coming up? A milestone birthday, a holiday, a wedding…even a breakup? Any shake-up in your routine can boost your quitting efforts.

93. Reward Yourself

Okay, you had all the pieces of your plan in place, and your quit date came around. You smoked your last cigarette, and you've been smoke-free…for a whole day. That's awesome! Think of small ways you can reward yourself for each day and week that you are smoke-free. The first few weeks after quitting are the hardest; after that the habit loop fades, and so do cravings.

Tips to Make the Habit Stick

- Cigarettes are expensive. Calculate how much you spent per day on smoking, and for every day you're smoke-free, deposit that amount in a piggy bank (or your savings account). In the US, for a pack-a-day smoker, this is $180 a month! Watch the money pile up. Think about how you'll spend it.

- Consider the health-related expenses of smoking and how much money you're saving yourself. In the US, this is $300 billion per year due to direct medical care costs and lost productivity. On an individual level, consider a heart attack, stroke, or cancer diagnosis. What would the doctor's visits and pharmacy co-pays be? If you stay quit, you're likely saving yourself from all that. That's probably worth a vacation somewhere really nice, at least.

- Cigarettes stink. Depending on how much you used to smoke, your clothes and living space may have that ashtray odor. (You don't notice this while you're smoking, but everyone else does.) If you feel confident about your quitting, trade your stinky old clothes for fresh new ones. Or do what a friend of mine did: redecorate your place. The smell of smoke will never come out of carpet and curtains. If you can, replace them, and enjoy your space.

94. Don't Gain Weight

Many people relapse into smoking because they gain weight when they quit. A big reason for this is the tendency to replace cigarettes with food. It's an oral habit thing. If you're aware of this, you can do something else and avoid the weight gain.

Tips to Make the Habit Stick

- Try chewing gum. This keeps your mouth busy and avoids calorie intake. Be aware that some sugarless gum contains sorbitol, which can cause gas.
- Have healthy snacks around. Good choices are foods that will occupy your jaws in a satisfying way, like crunchy carrot sticks and hot popcorn (plain or only lightly salted, of course).
- Go for a walk. This is a classic strategy for all cravings. A brisk walk down the hall, around the block, or even just to another room can disrupt the habit loop. Poof! Craving's gone. Bonus: you also got some activity.

95. Know Who You're Going to Call

You may need some assistance with quitting, and that's totally okay. Luckily, there is a lot of free assistance available for quitting smoking.

Tips to Make the Habit Stick

- The website www.smokefree.gov is an excellent resource with sections devoted to US military veterans, women, and people ages sixty and up, as well as Spanish speakers. It offers a live chat option as well as a free hotline. Consider checking it out: www.smokefree.gov/tools-tips/get-extra-help/speak-to-an-expert.
- There are apps for this. Free ones. Apps that will help you develop a plan and stay on track include QuitGuide and quitSTART. Find out about them at: www.smokefree.gov/tools-tips/apps.
- There's also a free text message program that will send you several friendly supportive text messages a day for six to eight weeks, the time when cravings are the strongest: www.smokefree.gov/smokefreetxt.

96. Consider Medications

Tobacco is a strongly addictive substance, and cigarettes are designed to make tobacco even more addictive. The brain reward pathways involved can make this heart-unhealthy habit very difficult to break. Medications can help disrupt the neurochemical pathway. Even benign, over-the-counter medications like nicotine replacement therapy (patches, gum, and lozenges) can double your chances of staying quit. Prescription medications bupropion, varenicline, and nortriptyline can have side effects but are considered safe and can be used along with nicotine replacement therapy.

Tips to Make the Habit Stick

- If you smoke daily, plan to use a combination of the patch and the gum or lozenges. The patch is long-acting and will reduce cravings overall. The gum or lozenges are for in-the-moment breakthrough cravings.

- If you smoke more than ten cigarettes per day, start with the highest-dose patch (21 mg/day) daily for at least six weeks, followed by the medium-dose patch (14 mg/day) for six weeks, followed by 7 mg/day for two weeks. If you smoke fewer than ten cigarettes per day, start with the medium-dose patch and go from there.

- Don't leave the patch on while you're sleeping and change the patch site daily to avoid skin irritation. (Smoking quit rates are the same whether the patch is left on for 24 hours or taken off at night.)

- Gum and lozenges are for cravings throughout the day. If morning nicotine cravings occur, put on your new patch and use the gum or lozenges while waiting for the new nicotine patch to take effect.

- For the nicotine gum, if you're smoking more than twenty-five cigarettes per day, use the 4-mg dose. If you smoke fewer than that, use the 2-mg dose. When cravings occur, chew one piece of gum for up to 30 minutes, up to twenty-four pieces of gum per day, for at least six weeks, and then taper off.
- If you have dental problems or use dentures, use nicotine lozenges. If you smoke within 30 minutes of awakening, you should use the 4-mg dose, but if you wait more than 30 minutes after awakening to smoke, use the 2-mg dose. Place a lozenge in your mouth for 30 minutes and let it melt. Use up to one lozenge every hour or two for six weeks, up to twenty lozenges per day, and then taper off.
- If patches, gum, and lozenges aren't working, consider talking to a doctor about prescription medications or explore additional options. The CDC's www.smokefree.gov website is a good source of additional information: www.smokefree.gov/tools-tips/how-to-quit/explore-quit-methods.

Alcohol Use Disorder

According to National Institutes of Health statistics, alcohol misuse is the fifth leading risk factor for premature death and disability in the world (and first for people aged fifteen to forty-nine). Alcohol is very habit forming, as well as addictive. As we learned in Chapter 5, a small amount of alcohol consumed regularly (up to seven drinks for women and up to fourteen drinks for men per week) is significantly associated with a lower risk of heart disease. However, anything over the recommended limit can actually cause heart and other medical problems (including alcohol use disorder), and is considered high-risk.

How do you know if you have alcohol use disorder? Here is a checklist based on the official diagnostic criteria.

Within the past year, have you:

- Had times when you ended up drinking more or longer than you intended?
- More than once wanted to cut down or stop drinking, or tried to, but couldn't? Spent a lot of time drinking? Or being sick or getting over the aftereffects?
- Experienced craving (a strong need, or urge, to drink)?
- Found that drinking (or being sick from drinking) often interfered with taking care of your home or family? Or caused job troubles? Or school problems?
- Continued to drink even though it was causing trouble with your family or friends?
- Given up or cut back on activities that used to be important or interesting to you, or were fun for you, in order to drink?
- More than once gotten into situations while drinking that increased your chances of getting hurt (such as driving, swimming, using machinery, walking in a dangerous area, or having unsafe sex)?
- Continued to drink even though it was making you feel depressed or anxious or adding to another health problem? Or after having had a memory blackout?
- Had to drink much more than you once did to get the effect you want? Or found that your usual number of drinks had much less effect than before?
- Found that when the effects of alcohol were wearing off, you had withdrawal symptoms, such as trouble sleeping, shakiness, irritability, anxiety, depression, restlessness, nausea, or sweating? Or sensed things that were not there?

If you have any two of these symptoms, your drinking is concerning and meets criteria for alcohol use disorder (having two or three is mild, four or five is moderate, and six or more is severe alcohol use disorder).

What should you do next? It's important to know that there are many treatment options available. But for some people with alcohol use disorder and alcohol dependence, suddenly quitting alcohol can be incredibly dangerous and even deadly. Sometimes a formal, medically supervised detoxification program is needed. For this reason, I'm not including habits here, because the best next step is to talk to a healthcare provider. If you want to learn more, the National Institute on Alcohol Abuse and Alcoholism has an excellent website with a free downloadable information packet and numerous alcohol assessment tools and tips, as well as links to other resources. This can all be found at www.rethinkingdrinking.niaaa.nih.gov/default.aspx.

Overeating

Many people struggle to control their eating habits, which can be a significant obstacle if they want to lose weight and live healthy. This may be due to underlying stress eating, binge eating disorder, or food addiction: all different behavioral problems with some overlap. Let's review each one to better understand what's behind the overeating, and then we'll discuss how to approach treatment.

Stress Eating

Stress eating is also referred to as *emotional* or *comfort eating*. We saw this in Chapter 3: eating unhealthy or large amounts of food in response to stress and negative emotions is a common unhealthy coping behavior. Stress eating is not a formal, official psychiatric or medical diagnosis; rather, it's a habit and potentially a heart-harmful one.

Case Study: Stress Eating

Shirley had a tough day at work, and she's feeling stressed and annoyed. She comes home for dinner and considers making herself a healthy meal, but nothing is prepped and she's tired. Now she's really craving something rich and comforting, like ice cream. Chocolate ice cream. She goes to the freezer and opens the container of ice cream, intending to only have a spoonful but ends up having a bowlful. "Oh well, I deserved it because I had a stressful day," she thinks.

Shirley's negative emotions trigger a craving for a comfort food: chocolate ice cream. She has the ice cream, and more than she intended, but she stops there and doesn't feel overly upset about it.

The Best Habits to Overcome Stress Eating

97. Pause and Reflect

If this type of stress eating is a pattern for you, just recognizing that is half the battle. In a study of ninety-nine overweight adults, providing nutrition education (on the Mediterranean diet) as well as emotional eating counseling resulted in weight loss of at least 10 percent total body weight for all participants. The authors concluded that once people recognize their coping strategy for negative emotions is eating unhealthy foods, they can learn better strategies.

Think about the last time you craved or ate something unhealthy. Was the trigger stress or another negative emotion? Then think about what might be a more effective (and healthier) coping strategy.

Tips to Make the Habit Stick

- Breathe. If you're feeling stressed, then do something proactive to relieve your stress. Tell your brain that you'll be right back to address that craving, but you're just going to do some deep breathing first. Try the Relaxation Response, even if just for three breaths.
- Call someone. If you had a stressful day, call a supportive friend or family member and talk it out.
- Distract your brain. Doing something else, anything else, in that moment can distract the brain from the craving and break the habit loop. Taking a little walk, even to another room, changes the environment and can sufficiently distract the craving brain (plus, it's exercise). Or, have a drink. Of water, or seltzer, or tea, that is. Often just putting something in your mouth will satisfy a craving, at least for a moment. Tea can be additionally comforting, and the moment may pass.

98. Be Prepared

If you know that you have a tendency toward stress eating, prepare ahead of time. There will always be stressful events. You may not always be able to avoid, manage, or distract yourself from them. How else can you be proactive if you have a tendency to stress eat?

Tips to Make the Habit Stick

- Don't buy the unhealthy foods that you tend to comfort-eat.
- If you buy these foods for others in your household, store them separately or even ask those family members to hide them.
- Have healthy, satisfying snacks around. Fresh cold fruit, or crunchy popcorn, or even frozen blueberries can trick the brain and quash that craving.
- Build a solid stress management routine into your daily schedule so that you aren't as affected when stuff happens.

Binge Eating Disorder

Binge eating disorder is a serious medical problem. It's increasingly common and yet was only recognized as a "real" diagnosis in 2015. In order to be diagnosed with binge eating disorder, someone has to have these formal criteria:

1. Binge eating that is recurrent and ongoing (at least once per week for at least three months)
2. Feeling upset and distressed about the binge eating
3. Binge eating that is associated with at least three of these:
   - Eating faster than normal
   - Eating until uncomfortably full

- Overeating even when not hungry
- Eating alone, out of embarrassment
- Feeling disgusted, ashamed, or depressed after overeating

4. No purging (inducing vomiting or abusing laxatives) after binge eating

(Note: purging after overeating is characteristic of bulimia, which is a separate eating disorder with a specific treatment approach.)

The trigger for the behavior is not always clear; rather, it's a recurring disorder that's very distressing, uncomfortable, and difficult to control. It's best treated by a team of providers, ideally including a physician or psychiatrist with experience in treating eating disorders, as well as a therapist and a registered dietitian.

I'm not including habits for this diagnosis or food addiction, because these really need to be addressed by medical professionals and can only respond to the appropriate treatment.

Food Addiction

Food addiction does not exist as a "real" psychiatric or medical diagnosis, and there is a lot of controversy around the concept. You may have seen news headlines like "Is Sugar Really As Addictive As Cocaine?" and "No, Sugar Isn't the New Heroin." This is because hard science looking at brain neurochemistry suggests that certain foods involve the same brain craving and reward pathways and are associated with the same behaviors as certain drugs. Some treatments mirror those of other addictions. Overeaters Anonymous is a twelve-step plan based on Alcoholics Anonymous and can be very helpful for people. Some medications overlap as well: naltrexone is used for opioid and alcohol use disorder. Contrave, a combination of naltrexone and bupropion, can be helpful in these situations as well.

Experts who argue against food addiction cite the fact that we need food to live, but we do not need alcohol and drugs. They also argue that foods don't cause physical dependence (as in needing more and more to get the same effect or having withdrawal symptoms after stopping).

It's important to point out that addictive foods tend to be human-invented, artificial, processed foods, which can act on the brain in a way similar to drugs, which are also human-invented, artificial, processed substances. Think about it. People don't struggle to control their consumption of apples and broccoli. They struggle with fast foods; fried foods; salty, crispy foods; sweet baked goods; sugary, creamy ice cream… heavily processed foods that do not exist in nature.

Regardless of how we label the problem, effective treatments exist and medical professionals should be involved.

Electronics Addiction

As we learned in Chapters 1 and 7, sitting for long periods of time is associated with increased risk of heart disease and increased risk of death from any cause. We also learned that sitting watching a screen is even worse for you. People know this, and yet they struggle to cut down on all kinds of screen time: TV viewing, Internet activities, video games, and smartphone use. The term *electronics addiction* comes to mind. While this does not yet exist as an official medical diagnosis, if you Google it, you'll see that a heck of a lot of people seem to be dealing with it.

Electronics overuse can have characteristics of other addictions and can be severe. People can feel compelled to use their device, despite negative physical and social consequences. Smartphones can be particularly problematic. In a 2017 UK survey of more than four thousand adults and teenagers, 79 percent checked their smartphones before falling asleep and more than 50 percent checked them within 15 minutes of waking. Even scarier: well over half look at their phones while walking! What's wrong with us?

As with other behavioral bad-habits-bordering-on-addiction, there is controversy over how to classify these disorders. Nevertheless, we can apply some healthy habit techniques to the problem.

99. Make It Harder to Use Your Device

No matter what device you're struggling with, you can make it inconvenient to use. This simple, logical trick can be very effective.

Tips to Make the Habit Stick

- Is it TV? Okay. Consider your TV issue and situation. If you have TVs in several rooms, pick one room that will be the designated media room and give the other TVs away. You don't need a TV in your kitchen or bedroom. Watching TV while eating is bad for you. Watching TV before bed is bad for you. Watching TV generally is bad for you. What's your conclusion?

- You can also roll your TV into a closet, unplug it, or hide the remote. This same strategy can apply to computers and gaming equipment.

- Have a healthy (and enjoyable!) backup activity that you can do instead. If it's gaming that's the issue, go for a run or to the gym. Play some pickup basketball, play with your kids, interact with people in real life and in a positive way. Is it nighttime Internet browsing? Nighttime is the perfect time to catch up on your reading list, or get in a few yoga poses, or meditate.

100. Take Advantage of Technology to Control Your Technology

If smartphone use is your issue, there are apps for that. A recent article in *The Guardian* reviewed a number of these. They're all a little different but generally work by helping you monitor your phone usage, keeping track of how much time you're wasting. They also ding you when you're on for too long. You can use your phone against itself!

If you get sidetracked by your social media and news alerts, you can turn them off. Same with the email notifications on your computer. You can also use the parental controls on your cable box to help you control your TV habit.

Tips to Make the Habit Stick

- Right now, check out some of these apps and consider trying one. You've got your phone on you, right? Space and Forest are both apps that make staying off your phone into a kind of a game, and they get high ratings. Moment and Mute are more shame-based. Flipd hides your apps from you. Try one or a few to see which work best for you.

- For most smartphones, you can turn off alerts by going to Settings and then Notifications. There will be a list of everything that can bleep and blink at you, and you can go through and swipe the "allow notifications" toggle to "off" for all of them.

- You can also choose not to use the technology on your phone. Set an old-fashioned alarm clock instead of using your phone alarm so you aren't tempted to look at it first thing in the morning.

Addressing Mental Health Can Lead to Physical Health

Addressing underlying mental health issues is critical to banishing bad habits and making heart-healthy lifestyle changes. Every healthcare provider with lifestyle change program experience I spoke to emphasized the need to address depression, anxiety, and stress first and foremost. In Chapter 2, we learned about cardiologist Dr. Malissa Wood, who developed a successful lifestyle change program for socioeconomically disadvantaged women by first asking her patients about their stress level. In Chapter 4, diabetes expert Dr. Stephanie Eisenstat described how important our emotional state is when it comes to adopting a healthy lifestyle. She emphasized: "If you're depressed and feeling overwhelmed, it's very hard to make any changes."

In one case, my middle-aged patient Sam started off with a BMI over 40, high blood pressure, and high cholesterol, but over the course of a year she lost over 100 pounds to a BMI of 27, and got her blood pressure and cholesterol to normal. How did she do it? She describes her multipronged treatment approach, which involved medications, Overeaters Anonymous (OA), and habit change: "I absolutely believe that I was suffering from depression, but hadn't reached out for help until I was at my wits' end." Now, "even if every day is not a perfect, totally healthy, clean eating day, I still feel a million times better than before I started medication." OA was also critical: "OA reminds me that I'm not like everyone else in terms of my eating. I'm a food addict, and I can't trick myself into thinking I'm cured. I'll always be struggling with food issues. I have to remember that I need to stay vigilant." As far as habits, "I didn't attempt to change them all at once. I figured that all of my bad habits were what got me to my heaviest weight, so trying to eliminate even the smallest bad habit, one at a time, would make a difference, which it did." These all have helped this patient stay emotionally stable. "I don't spiral out like I used to. Which is huge. If I don't have a great eating day, I still get up the next day and feel positive that it's a new day, and I have the ability to move on."

Like many others who have made positive life changes, this patient is taking it one day at a time, for life.

Consider and Address Your Own Mental Health Issues

Is it possible that your mood is sabotaging your heart-health efforts? Mental health factors can make lifestyle change difficult. Underlying depression and anxiety may need to be addressed and treated. Take these two diagnostic quizzes to see what your scores are.

Following is the Patient Health Questionnaire depression module, a widely used questionnaire to screen for and monitor depression.

A score of 1–4 indicates minimal depression; 5–9 signals mild depression; 10–14 is moderate; 15–19 shows moderately severe; and 20–27 indicates severe depression. A score over 10 is indicative of a depression diagnosis, and any positive response to the last question is concerning. Please, if you are in either of these categories, talk to your doctor or a mental health professional.

PATIENT HEALTH QUESTIONNAIRE-9 (PHQ-9)

Over the <u>last 2 weeks</u>, how often have you been bothered by any of the following problems? *(Use "✔" to indicate your answer)*	Not at all	Several days	More than half the days	Nearly every day
1. Little interest or pleasure in doing things	0	1	2	3
2. Feeling down, depressed, or hopeless	0	1	2	3
3. Trouble falling or staying asleep, or sleeping too much	0	1	2	3
4. Feeling tired or having little energy	0	1	2	3
5. Poor appetite or overeating	0	1	2	3
6. Feeling bad about yourself — or that you are a failure or have let yourself or your family down	0	1	2	3
7. Trouble concentrating on things, such as reading the newspaper or watching television	0	1	2	3
8. Moving or speaking so slowly that other people could have noticed? Or the opposite — being so fidgety or restless that you have been moving around a lot more than usual	0	1	2	3
9. Thoughts that you would be better off dead or of hurting yourself in some way	0	1	2	3

FOR OFFICE CODING ___0___ + _____ + _____ + _____

=Total Score: _____

If you checked off <u>any</u> problems, how <u>difficult</u> have these problems made it for you to do your work, take care of things at home, or get along with other people?

Not difficult at all	Somewhat difficult	Very difficult	Extremely difficult
☐	☐	☐	☐

Developed by Drs. Robert L. Spitzer, Janet B.W. Williams, Kurt Kroenke and colleagues, with an educational grant from Pfizer Inc. No permission required to reproduce, translate, display or distribute.

Following is the Generalized Anxiety Disorder Questionnaire, widely used to screen for and monitor anxiety. Take it and check your level of anxiety. If it's high, look at some habits to bring it down.

A score of 1–4 shows minimal anxiety; 5–9 indicates mild; 10–14 shows moderate; and 15 and over shows severe anxiety. A score over 10 is fairly indicative of an anxiety diagnosis, so if you scored over 10, please talk to your doctor or a mental health professional.

GAD-7

Over the <u>last 2 weeks</u>, how often have you been bothered by the following problems? *(Use "✔" to indicate your answer)*	Not at all	Several days	More than half the days	Nearly every day
1. Feeling nervous, anxious or on edge	0	1	2	3
2. Not being able to stop or control worrying	0	1	2	3
3. Worrying too much about different things	0	1	2	3
4. Trouble relaxing	0	1	2	3
5. Being so restless that it is hard to sit still	0	1	2	3
6. Becoming easily annoyed or irritable	0	1	2	3
7. Feeling afraid as if something awful might happen	0	1	2	3

(For office coding: Total Score T____ = ____ + ____ + ____)

Developed by Drs. Robert L. Spitzer, Janet B.W. Williams, Kurt Kroenke and colleagues, with an educational grant from Pfizer Inc. No permission required to reproduce, translate, display or distribute.

Most importantly if you feel as if you may have depression, anxiety, or a different mental health issue, please ask a doctor or mental health professional for help. While a healthy diet and lifestyle is a big part of any treatment strategy, therapy and/or medications may be necessary as well.

Talk to Someone

If you feel depressed or stressed, overwhelmed, or anxious, then please talk to a healthcare provider about your feelings. There are questions they can ask to sort out what might be going on, and there are a variety of treatment options. Some people do well with therapy, others need medications, some need both, and all need good self-care. Talk to your doctor about how you feel or check out the websites listed in Chapter 4 to connect with a mental health professional. For anyone with severe depression, especially thoughts of ending their life, the National Suicide Prevention Lifeline (https://suicidepreventionlifeline.org/) is a toll-free phone call that can connect you to a caring, trained professional who can listen and help you connect to the right resources: 1-800-273-TALK (8255).

In this chapter you've learned about how habit and addiction can overlap, how to recognize certain addictions and approach some common heart-unhealthy habits, and when you may need additional help managing underlying mental health issues.

In summary, lifestyle change is not easy, but with a solid understanding of how bad habits are broken and good habits are formed, plus plenty of evidence-based medical advice, you can transform yourself. The next section includes heart-healthy recipes, designed to be simple, fast, budget-friendly, and low-tech.

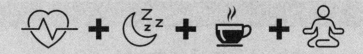

Appendix A

Recipes

YOU'VE SEEN THESE tantalizing recipe ideas scattered throughout Chapters 5 and 6. These recipes were developed with input from Boston-area farm-to-table Chef de Cuisine Cassidy Salus. None require special equipment or hard-to-find ingredients.

Nutrition information per serving is provided, calculated using the Verywell Fit Recipe Analyzer (which you can use for your recipes as well, at www.verywellfit.com/recipe-nutrition-analyzer-4157076).

Let's eat!

Beverages

Bubbly Minty Mojito Mocktail
Gluten-free, vegan, no sodium

Whether you're cutting down on alcohol or simply trying to drink more water, this healthy, light take on a favorite cocktail will make it easier.

Serves 4
1 cup fresh mint leaves, rinsed very well
3 limes, sliced into thin wedges
Ice to preference
1 liter lime seltzer (no sodium added)

1. Put the mint leaves at the bottom of a pitcher.
2. Using a wooden spoon, squish the mint up a bit. It doesn't have to be pulverized—the goal is to release the minty essence without everyone getting little green bits in their teeth.
3. Add the lime wedges and ice.
4. Pour the seltzer over the ice.
5. Stir lightly.
6. Serve in tall glasses.

Per serving: Calories: 0 | Fat: 0 | Protein: 0 | Sodium: 0 | Carbohydrates: 0 | Fiber: 0 | Sugar: 0

Breakfasts

Filling Fruit and Nut Bowl with Greek Yogurt
Gluten-free, low sodium

You can get in two or more servings of fruits at breakfast alone. This is my standard breakfast. I use organic mixed frozen berries that we buy in 3-pound bags from the bulk grocery store, and I feel great about getting all those antioxidants and fiber first thing. Adding cinnamon tastes great, and evidence suggests that ground cinnamon lowers blood sugars. Greek yogurt is particularly full of goodness, including gut-healthy probiotics. This breakfast recipe is meant to be versatile and personalized. If this is not a filling enough breakfast for you, add more nuts, seeds, or toasted oats. Note: A version of this recipe was published on *Harvard Health Blog*.

Serves 1
2 cups mixed berries (fresh or frozen, but unsweetened)
$\frac{1}{4}$ cup sliced almonds
1 teaspoon cinnamon
$\frac{1}{2}$ cup plain, low-fat Greek yogurt

1. Add the fruit, nuts, and cinnamon to a medium bowl or travel container.
2. Enjoy with plain Greek yogurt on top or alongside.

Per serving: Calories: 390 | Fat: 14.4g | Saturated Fat: 2.1g | Protein: 14g | Sodium: 86mg | Carbohydrates: 49.6g | Fiber: 14.2g | Sugars: 29.7g | Calcium: 351mg | Iron: 3mg | Potassium: 831mg

Overnight Oats
Gluten-free, low sodium

Oatmeal in the morning is a cinch with these recipes you prepare the night before. If you want to heat them up, use a microwave-safe container.

Cherry Chocolate Overnight Oats

Chocolate and cherries just naturally go together and complement one another's deliciousness. This is a great way to start the day!

Serves 1
$\frac{1}{2}$ **cup gluten-free oats (rolled)**
$\frac{1}{2}$ **cup boiling water**
$\frac{1}{2}$ **cup frozen cherries**
$\frac{1}{2}$ **cup unsweetened non-dairy milk (I use almond milk)**
$\frac{1}{4}$ **cup dark chocolate bits (at least 60 percent cacao)**

1. Pour the oats and boiling water in a medium-sized travel container.
2. Put the frozen cherries and non-dairy milk on top.
3. Cover and let sit in refrigerator overnight.
4. When you're ready to eat, if you'd like it hot, microwave for 30–60 seconds. Stir.
5. Add the dark chocolate on top and enjoy!

Per serving: Calories: 327 | Fat: 9.2g | Saturated Fat: 3.3g | Protein: 11g | Sodium: 69mg | Carbohydrates: 54g | Fiber: 6.1g | Sugars: 20.3g | Calcium: 66mg | Iron: 3mg | Potassium: 390mg

Apple Cinnamon Walnut Overnight Oats

Serves 1

$1/2$ cup gluten-free oats (rolled)
$1/2$ cup boiling water
$1/2$ cup chopped apple (about 1 small apple)
$1/2$ teaspoon cinnamon
2 tablespoons chopped walnuts
$1/2$ cup non-dairy milk (I use almond milk)

1. Pour the oats and boiling water in a travel container.
2. Put the chopped apple, cinnamon, walnuts, and milk on top.
3. Cover and let sit in refrigerator overnight.
4. When you're ready to eat, if you'd like it hot, microwave for 30–60 seconds. Stir and enjoy!

Per serving: Calories: 378 | Fat: 14.2g | Saturated Fat: 1.2g | Protein: 13.5g | Sodium: 70mg | Carbohydrates: 53g | Fiber: 9.2g | Sugars: 17g | Calcium: 77mg | Iron: 4mg | Potassium: 500mg

Appetizers

Almost Homemade Corn Tortilla Chips with Black Bean Salsamole
Gluten-free, vegan

This is a healthier take on a popular appetizer. Take advantage of quality corn tortillas, jarred or freshly prepared low-sodium salsa, and unsalted canned beans from the grocery store. Look for salsa with less than 100 mg of sodium per 2-tablespoon serving. Trader Joe's, Newman's Own, and Muir Glen all make versions. The salsa-bean-guacamole combo is always a hit at gatherings, and people will think you worked a lot harder than you did!

Serves 8

Almost Homemade Corn Tortilla Chips
1 package of regular-sized (6-inch) corn tortillas, usually 8 to a package (made without lard)
1 tablespoon extra-virgin olive oil, for brushing

Black Bean Salsamole
1½ cups low-sodium salsa
1 (15.5-ounce) can unsalted black beans
1 ripe avocado, cut into small cubes
2 tablespoons fresh lime juice

1. *For Almost Homemade Corn Tortilla Chips:* Preheat oven to 375°F.
2. Lightly brush each of the tortillas with a small amount of olive oil.
3. Using kitchen scissors, cut the tortillas into 6 triangles each (for 48 triangles total).

4. Spread half of the triangles out onto a large baking sheet and put into the oven.
5. Bake for 4–6 minutes, until browned. Remove from oven and allow to cool.
6. Repeat for other half of triangles.
7. Serve or store, covered, for up to two days.
8. *For Black Bean Salsamole:* Gently mix all ingredients together in a medium serving bowl. Serve alongside chips.

Per serving: Calories: 153 | Fat: 7.6g | Saturated Fat: 1.4g | Protein: 3.9g | Sodium: 162mg | Carbohydrates: 19.7g | Fiber: 5.3g | Sugars: 2.1g | Calcium: 40mg | Iron: 1mg | Potassium: 365mg

Salads

Nutty Tabbouleh Salad
Vegan, low sodium

My version of this classic Middle Eastern salad takes advantage of arugula's natural pepperiness, which is balanced out by the warm comfort of whole grains and crunchy toasted almonds. The almonds add protein and healthy fat, making this a heartier salad that's also good for your heart.

Serves 6 (as side salad)

Dressing

4 tablespoons lemon juice
4 tablespoons extra-virgin olive oil
2 garlic cloves, crushed and finely chopped
$\frac{1}{4}$ teaspoon salt
$\frac{1}{2}$ teaspoon black pepper
$\frac{1}{2}$ teaspoon dried oregano

Salad

1 cup uncooked bulgur (cracked wheat) (makes 2 cups cooked)
2 cups water
1 cup sliced almonds, unsalted
6 cups arugula, rinsed
2 cups diced fresh tomatoes
1 cup diced fresh cucumber
$\frac{1}{4}$ cup peeled and finely chopped red onion

1. *For the Dressing:* Whisk all ingredients together in a small bowl.
2. *For the Salad:* Put the bulgur and water into a small saucepan and bring to a simmer for 5 minutes, then cover and let sit. This can be done ahead and the bulgur left to cool.
3. To toast the almonds, heat a small frying pan over low heat, then add the almonds. Heat, shaking the pan occasionally, until just fragrant and very lightly browned (2–3 minutes).
4. In a large salad bowl, toss arugula, tomatoes, cucumber, onion, almonds, and cooked bulgur together. This can be covered and stored in the refrigerator for up to a day.
5. Just before serving, add dressing and mix well.

Per serving: Calories: 274 | Fat: 18g | Saturated Fat: 2.1g | Protein: 7.3g | Sodium: 115mg | Carbohydrates: 25.6g | Fiber: 7.5g | Sugars: 3.3g | Calcium: 84mg | Iron: 2mg | Potassium: 445mg

Summer Corn, Tomato, Spinach, and Basil Salad
Gluten-free, vegan, low sodium

Yes, corn kernels are whole grains! Using frozen corn niblets makes this light summer salad a breeze, but go ahead and let your friends think you spent a ton of time shucking ears of corn and then removing the kernels by hand. I won't tell. This salad is especially good with grilled food.

Serves 6 (as side salad)

Dressing

$\frac{1}{8}$ cup white wine vinegar
$\frac{1}{4}$ cup olive oil
2 garlic cloves, crushed and minced fine (1 teaspoon)
$\frac{1}{4}$ teaspoon salt
$\frac{1}{2}$ teaspoon black pepper
$\frac{1}{2}$ teaspoon dried oregano

Salad

4 cups plain frozen corn niblets
$\frac{1}{4}$ cup water
2 cups diced tomatoes
1 cup washed and roughly chopped fresh basil
8 cups baby spinach leaves, washed (about two 6-ounce packages)

1. *For the Dressing:* Whisk all ingredients together in a small bowl.
2. *For the Salad:* Put the corn in a microwave-safe bowl and add the ¼ cup of water. Cook on high for 1 minute, then stir. Cook for another 2 minutes until niblets are tender. Allow corn to cool. This can be done a day ahead and the corn stored in the refrigerator.
3. In a large salad bowl, toss cooled cooked corn, tomatoes, basil, and spinach.
4. Just before serving, add dressing and toss well to coat.

Per serving: Calories: 214 | Fat: 10g | Saturated Fat: 1.5g | Protein: 5.5g | Sodium: 115mg | Carbohydrates: 32g | Fiber: 4g | Sugars: 5.3g | Iron: 2mg | Potassium: 621mg

Niçoise-Style Sardine Salad
Gluten-free

This is a colorful, crowd-pleasing, budget-friendly, heart-healthy salad. The idea is to arrange each ingredient on a serving platter so that people can pick and choose what they want, like a mini salad bar (one that features plenty of plant nutrients and omega-3 PUFAs). You don't need oil or salt in the dressing, because you're using the oil drained from the sardines, which has more omega-3 PUFAs than the sardines themselves—double, in fact!

Serves 6 (as an appetizer salad)

Dressing

$\frac{1}{8}$ cup white wine vinegar
The oil drained from 2 cans of sardines
2 tablespoons Dijon mustard
$\frac{1}{2}$ teaspoon black pepper
3 tablespoons chopped fresh dill

Salad

$\frac{1}{2}$ pound assorted small potatoes, quartered, red/purple/yellow mix ideal
2 cups trimmed green beans
1 head romaine lettuce, chopped
2 cups halved cherry tomatoes
2 cups peeled, shredded carrots
1 cup radishes, sliced thinly
2 (4.4-ounce) cans sardines, drained (the oil goes into the dressing, so don't throw it away!)
$\frac{1}{4}$ cup Niçoise olives (regular black olives are fine as well)

1. *For the Dressing:* Whisk all ingredients together in a small bowl and set aside.
2. *For the Salad:* Fill a medium-sized saucepan with enough water to cover the potatoes and put in the potatoes. Bring to a boil and then turn down to a simmer. Boil for 4–6 minutes, until fork-tender. Remove the potatoes using a slotted spoon and let cool. Put the green beans into the simmering water and cook for 3–5 minutes, until tender. Remove and let cool.
3. Spread the romaine lettuce over a platter.
4. Arrange the tomatoes, carrots, radishes, green beans, potatoes, and sardines in "stripes" or piles on the platter. Scatter your olives over and around the vegetables and sardines (or in their own area if you prefer).
5. Drizzle dressing over the salad and serve.

Per serving: Calories: 215 | Fat: 12.1g | Saturated Fat: 2.7g | Protein: 10.5g | Sodium: 310mg | Carbohydrates: 17.6g | Fiber: 4.9g | Sugars: 4.5g | Vitamin D: 106mg | Calcium: 197mg | Iron: 4mg | Potassium: 727mg

Soups

Superfood Lentil Soup
Gluten-free, vegan

Red lentils cook fast, unlike the green and brown varieties. Lentils are also amazingly good for you, as are colorful peppers, spinach, and antioxidant spices like ginger and turmeric. Use plain water for the base so you can control the amount of salt that goes into your soup. Garlic and ginger can be bought pre-chopped in jars or as a paste in tubes, which can make cooking so much easier. If you also have frozen spinach, then this meal is easy.

Serves 6

2 tablespoons extra-virgin olive oil
$\frac{1}{2}$ onion, peeled and chopped small
1 cup finely diced red peppers
2 cloves garlic, crushed and minced (or a teaspoon of garlic paste)
1" piece of ginger, peeled and grated (or a teaspoon of ginger paste)
6 cups water
2 cups red lentils
1 cup chopped spinach, frozen, unsalted
$\frac{1}{2}$ teaspoon salt
$\frac{1}{2}$ teaspoon pepper
$\frac{1}{2}$ teaspoon turmeric
$\frac{1}{2}$ teaspoon red pepper flakes
4 tablespoons lemon juice

1. Heat olive oil in a large soup pot set over medium heat.
2. Add the onion and peppers, and sauté until soft, about 2–3 minutes.
3. Add the garlic and ginger, and sauté until fragrant, another minute.
4. Add the water and bring to a simmer.
5. Add the lentils, spinach, salt, pepper, turmeric, and red pepper flakes and let simmer for 3–5 minutes, until lentils and spinach are tender. Then turn off the heat.
6. Just before serving, add lemon juice, stir, and serve.

Per serving: Calories: 285 | Fat: 5.6g | Saturated Fat: 0.8g | Protein: 17.4g | Sodium: 212mg | Carbohydrates: 42.5g | Fiber: 20.4g | Sugars: 3g | Potassium: 755mg

Antioxidant Chili
Gluten-free, vegan

This plant-nutrient powerhouse chili is also deliciously decadent, featuring colorful carrots, peppers, and fire-roasted tomatoes, fiber- and protein-filled legumes, polyphenol-packed dark chocolate and herbs, and resveratrol-rich red wine. It's reminiscent of a Mexican mole sauce but much easier to make. Though this chili has a lot of ingredients, many are already in your pantry, and they all go into one pot.

Serves 8

1 tablespoon extra-virgin olive oil
1 small peeled yellow onion, grated or chopped fine
2 cloves garlic, crushed and minced (or 1 teaspoon of garlic paste)
$\frac{1}{2}$ cup red wine
1 large peeled carrot, grated

1 red bell pepper, diced small
1 yellow bell pepper, diced small
2 (16-ounce) cans diced fire-roasted tomatoes (and liquid)
$3\frac{1}{2}$ cups water
2 tablespoons dark 100 percent cocoa powder (like Ghirardelli)
3 teaspoons chili powder
1 teaspoon paprika
2 teaspoons cumin
$\frac{1}{4}$ teaspoon salt
$\frac{1}{2}$ teaspoon black pepper
$\frac{1}{2}$ teaspoon garlic powder
$\frac{1}{2}$ teaspoon onion powder
$\frac{1}{2}$ teaspoon cinnamon
$\frac{1}{2}$ teaspoon cayenne pepper
4 (16-ounce) cans no-salt-added beans
4 tablespoons lemon juice
1 cup cilantro, rinsed well and chopped
1 avocado, cubed

1. Heat the olive oil over medium heat and add onion and garlic.
2. Sauté until very soft, then add wine, stirring for 1–2 minutes.
3. Add carrots and peppers and stir, cooking until soft.
4. Add the tomatoes, water, cocoa powder and all the spices, stirring to combine. Then add the beans and simmer on low heat for 1 hour.
5. Add the lemon juice and cilantro before serving, reserving a few teaspoons of cilantro.
6. Serve with cubed avocado and extra cilantro sprinkled over.

Per serving: Calories: 346 | Fat: 8.3g | Saturated Fat: 1.7g | Protein: 17.3g | Sodium: 196mg | Carbohydrates: 51g | Fiber: 19.3g | Sugars: 4.1g | Calcium: 113mg | Iron: 5mg | Potassium: 134mg

Mains

Secret Ingredient Baltimore-Style Salmon Patties with Not-Oily Aioli
Gluten-free

This is a family favorite, and no one knows that it features super-nutritious puréed pumpkin! Most salmon cake recipes call for eggs and bread crumbs as binders, but puréed pumpkin and grated carrot work just as well, lend beautiful color, and add plenty of fiber and plant nutrients. Canned salmon is way cheaper than fresh and has just as much omega-3 PUFAs and calcium. Serve this alongside a salad (the Summer Corn, Tomato, Spinach, and Basil Salad would go perfectly) for a well-rounded meal.

Serves 4 (1 large patty each)

Secret Ingredient Baltimore-Style Salmon Patties

1 (15-ounce) can pink salmon, no salt added

$\frac{1}{2}$ cup puréed pumpkin

$\frac{1}{2}$ cup grated carrot (I use a handheld box grater.)

2 tablespoons minced chives (Don't have chives? Minced green onions or any onions will do.)

2 teaspoons Old Bay Seasoning

1 tablespoon olive oil

$\frac{1}{2}$ large lemon, sliced, for serving

Not-Oily Aioli

$\frac{1}{2}$ cup plain low-fat Greek yogurt
Juice and zest from $\frac{1}{2}$ a large lemon
1 clove garlic, crushed and minced fine
2 tablespoons chopped fresh dill

1. *For the Patties:* Mix all ingredients for the salmon patties together in a medium bowl.
2. Form patties with your hands and set on a plate or tray (you should have 4 burger-sized patties).
3. Heat oil in a large skillet over medium heat.
4. Set patties in skillet and brown for 4 minutes, then carefully flip.
5. Brown the other side, then serve hot.
6. *For the Aioli:* Mix all ingredients for the aioli together in a small bowl.
7. Plop a dollop alongside or on top of each salmon patty and serve with a slice of lemon.

Per serving: Calories: 367 | Fat: 13.6g | Saturated Fat: 4.4g | Protein: 46g | Sodium: 519mg | Carbohydrates: 13.2g | Fiber: 1.3g | Sugars: 9g | Calcium: 505mg | Iron: 1mg | Potassium: 696mg

Super-Simple Cashew Stir-Fry
Gluten-free, vegan

We make this basic recipe *a lot* in our home. I can attest to the fact that preparation can take fewer than 10 minutes total. Using frozen unseasoned veggies, garlic and ginger in tubes, plus cashews from the pantry makes this a very fast, easy, healthy meal option. Serve alongside brown rice for a heartier meal.

Serves 4
2 tablespoons sesame oil
1 teaspoon garlic paste
2 teaspoons ginger paste
7 cups unseasoned frozen stir-fry vegetables (two 10.8-ounce bags)
2 tablespoons low-sodium soy sauce
$\frac{1}{2}$ cup raw, unsalted cashews
3 cups cooked brown rice (for serving)

1. Heat a skillet or wok over medium-high heat.
2. Add the sesame oil, garlic, and ginger, stirring until fragrant.
3. Add vegetables and soy sauce, and stir.
4. Cover and let vegetables steam for 3–5 minutes.
5. Top with cashews and serve alongside heated brown rice.

Per serving: Calories: 341 | Fat: 15.5g | Saturated Fat: 2.6g | Protein: 7.3g | Sodium: 256mg | Carbohydrates: 42.1g | Fiber: 6g | Sugars: 5.6g | Iron: 4mg | Potassium: 537mg

Desserts

Dark Chocolate–Dipped Strawberries
Gluten-free, low sodium

Dark chocolate and berries combined make a decadent dessert, but you can feel good about it because both are rich in plant nutrients that help heal damage to your blood vessels and keep your heart healthy. (Note: A version of this recipe was published on *Harvard Health Blog*.)

Serves 6 (2 large strawberries each)

12 large fresh strawberries

1³⁄₄ cups dark chocolate pieces (You can use chopped chocolate bars or packaged chips. I use dark chocolate chips, which are 60 percent cacao, and one 10-ounce bag is about 1³⁄₄ cups.)

1 teaspoon canola oil (Almond, walnut, or hazelnut oil will lend a lovely flavor, but canola oil is fine.)

1. Wash and thoroughly dry the berries. (The chocolate sticks better when they're very dry.) Do not remove the caps.

2. Pour the chocolate pieces into a medium-sized microwave-safe mixing bowl and add the oil.

3. Place the bowl in the microwave and heat on high for 30 seconds. Remove and stir. The only thing melted will be the oil.

4. Microwave again for 30 seconds and stir. Repeat twice, until most pieces are melted. If there are only a few small chunks left, stir for a minute and see if they melt without any further microwaving. Chocolate burns very, very easily, and it tastes awful when it does.

5. Place a piece of parchment or wax paper on a baking sheet.

6. Gently grasp a berry by the green cap and lower into the chocolate "bath." Use a spoon to push chocolate up each berry until it is coated. Let excess chocolate drip off.
7. Place each berry onto the paper-covered baking sheet.
8. Place the baking sheet of berries in the fridge or in another cool place. Let the chocolate harden into a shell; this may take only a few minutes.
9. These will last about a day covered in the refrigerator.
10. If you have leftover chocolate, drop 2" round dollops onto the parchment or wax paper and save for later.

Per serving: Calories: 193 | Fat: 13.8g | Saturated Fat: 7.8g | Protein: 2.5g | Sodium: 5mg | Carbohydrates: 20.5g | Fiber: 5.2g | Sugars: 15.1g | Iron: 2mg | Potassium: 244mg

Orange Pistachio Dark Chocolate Bark
Gluten-free, low sodium

Both dark chocolate and nuts are especially heart-healthy. This simple dessert is perfect to serve to guests after dinner with tea and coffee.

Serves 8

1¾ cups dark chocolate pieces (You can use chopped chocolate bars or packaged chips. I use dark chocolate chips, which are 60 percent cacao, and one 10-ounce bag is about 1¾ cups.)
1 teaspoon canola oil (Almond, walnut, hazelnut, or extra-virgin olive oil is fine.)
½ cup crushed unsalted pistachios, raw
The zest of one medium orange

1. Pour the chocolate pieces into a medium-sized microwave-safe mixing bowl.
2. Add oil and stir it into the chocolate pieces.
3. Place bowl in microwave and heat on high for no more than 30 seconds at a time, stirring after each time, until chocolate is melted. Do not burn chocolate.
4. Pour onto a cookie sheet or baking pan that has been fitted with a silicone baking mat or nonstick parchment paper. Spread the chocolate out so that it's about ⅛" thick.
5. Sprinkle crushed nuts and orange zest over, and set pan in a cool place until bark is hardened.
6. Break into irregular pieces. Bark will last a few days wrapped in plastic or wax paper.

Per serving: Calories: 220 | Fat: 16.6g | Saturated Fat: 8.9g | Protein: 3.3g | Sodium: 5mg | Carbohydrates: 20.7g | Fiber: 5.2g | Sugars: 15.2g | Iron: 3mg | Potassium: 213mg

Appendix B

References

Chapter 1

Heart disease is... "Cardiovascular Disease," The World Health Organization, www.who.int/ cardiovascular_diseases/en/. Accessed April 2018.

In the United States... and Heart disease is often... "Heart Disease Facts," Centers for Disease Control and Prevention, updated November 28, 2017, www.cdc .gov/heartdisease/facts.htm.

People with diabetes... W.D. Strain and P.M. Paldánius, "Diabetes, Cardiovascular Disease, and the Microcirculation," Cardiovascular Diabetology 17(1):57, 2018.

Microvascular disease... Y. Shi and J.M. Wardlaw, "Update on Cerebral Small Vessel Disease: A Dynamic Whole Brain Disease," Stroke and Vascular Neurology 1(3), 2016, pp. 83–92.

There is a new medical term... E.A. Leonard and R.J. Marshall, "Cardiovascular Disease in Women," Primary Care: Clinics in Office Practice 45, 2018, pp. 131–141.

Strokes kill 6.7 million... "Cardiovascular Disease," The World Health Organization, www.who.int/cardiovascular_ diseases/en/. Accessed April 2018.

African Americans tend... "African Americans and Heart Disease, Stroke," American Heart Association, updated July 31, 2015, www.heart.org/ HEARTORG/conditions/more/ myheartandstrokenews/african- americans-and-heart-disease- stroke_UCM_444863_article .jsp#.WvBueTMh1aQ.

Native Americans, Latinos, and... "Race and Ethnicity: Clues to Your Heart Disease Risk?," Harvard Heart Letter, updated July 17, 2015, www.health .harvard.edu/heart-health/race- and-ethnicity-clues-to-your-heart- disease-risk.

Research shows that racial... "Health, United States, 2015: With Special Feature on Racial and Ethnic Health Disparities," National Center for Health Statistics, updated June 22, 2017, www.cdc.gov/nchs/data/hus/ hus15.pdf.

Studies suggest... R.R. Hardeman et al., "Structural Racism and Supporting Black Lives—The Role of Health Professionals," The New England Journal of Medicine 375, 1 December 2016, pp. 2,113–2,115.

Heart disease is the... M. Garcia et al., "Cardiovascular Disease in Women," Circulation Research 118, 15 April 2016, pp. 1,273–1,293.

2017 guidelines... and A 20-point higher... P.K. Whelton et al., "2017 Guideline for the Prevention, Detection, Evaluation, and Management of High Blood Pressure in Adults: Executive Summary," Journal of the American College of Cardiology, 2017 pp. 352–353.

The LDL, or bad... B. Ference et al., "Low-Density Lipoproteins Cause Atherosclerotic Cardiovascular Disease," European Heart Journal 38(32), 21 August 2017, pp. 2,459–2,472 and M. Feng et al., "Impact of Lipoproteins on Atherobiology," Cardiology Clinics 36(2), May 2018, pp. 193–201.

We now understand... G. Vannice and H. Rasmussen, "Position of the Academy of Nutrition and Dietetics: Dietary Fatty Acids for Healthy Adults," Journal of the Academy of Nutrition and Dietetics 114(1), January 2014, pp. 136–153.

People who have diabetes and Type 2 diabetes is not only... N. Sarwar et al., "Diabetes Mellitus, Fasting Blood Glucose Concentration, and Risk of Vascular Disease," The Lancet 375, 26 June 2010, pp. 2,215–2,222 and S.M. Haffner et al., "Mortality from Coronary Heart Disease in Subjects with Type 2 Diabetes and in Nondiabetic Subjects with and Without Myocardial Infarction," The New England Journal of Medicine 339, 23 July 1998, pp. 229–234.

In a large study... The DPP Research Group: The Diabetes Prevention Program (DPP): Description of a Lifestyle Intervention. *Diabetes Care* 25(12), 2002, pp. 2,165–2,171.

Being obese... and *An analysis of fifty-four studies...* C. Ma et al., "Effects of Weight Loss Interventions for Adults Who Are Obese on Mortality, Cardiovascular Disease, and Cancer," *The BMJ* 359, 14 November 2017, J4849.

Losing even just... L. Moore et al., "Can Sustained Weight Loss in Overweight Individuals Reduce the Risk of Diabetes Mellitus?," *Epidemiology* 11, May 2000, pp. 269–273.

This is called... S.G. Wannamethee and J.L. Atkins, "Muscle Loss and Obesity: The Health Implications of Sarcopenia and Sarcopenic Obesity," *The Proceedings of the Nutrition Society* 74(4), November 2015, pp. 405–412.

Having three or more... A. Galassi et al., "Metabolic Syndrome and Risk of Cardiovascular Disease: A Meta-analysis," *The American Journal of Medicine* 119(10), October 2006, pp. 812–819.

Having depression... D.L. Hare et al., "Depression and Cardiovascular Disease: A Clinical Review," *European Heart Journal* 35(21), 1 June 2014, pp. 1,365–1,372 and M.A. Whooley and J.M. Wong, "Depression and Cardiovascular Disorders," *Annual Review of Clinical Psychology* 9, 2013, pp. 327–354.

OSA is... T. Kendzerska et al., "Obstructive Sleep Apnea and Risk of Cardiovascular Events and All-Cause Mortality: A Decade-Long Historical Cohort Study," *PLoS Medicine* 11, 4 February 2014, p. e1001599 and L.F. Drager LF et al., "Sleep Apnea and Cardiovascular Disease," *Circulation* 136(19), 7 November 2017, pp. 1,840–1,850.

A diet high in refined... B. Dieter and K. Tuttle, "Dietary Strategies for Cardiovascular Health," *Trends in Cardiovascular Medicine* 27, July 2017, pp. 295–313.

Mountains of evidence... X. Wang et al., "Red and Processed Meat Consumption and Mortality: Dose-Response Meta-analysis of Prospective Cohort Studies," *Public Health Nutrition* 19(5), April 2016, pp. 895–905 and A. Wolk, "Potential Health Hazards of Eating Red Meat," *Journal of Internal Medicine* 281(2), February 2017, pp. 106–122.

Eating red meat... S. Tian et al., "Dietary Protein Consumption and the Risk of Type 2 Diabetes: A Systematic Review and Meta-analysis of Cohort Studies," *Nutrients* 9(9), 6 September 2017, p. 982.

Saturated fats are... L. Hooper et al., "Reduction in Saturated Fat Intake for Cardiovascular Disease," *The Cochrane Database of Systematic Reviews* (6), 10 June 2015, CD011737.

It is very well established... "Physical Inactivity," World Health Organization, www .who.int/dietphysicalactivity/ factsheet_inactivity/en/. Accessed May 2018.

Being inactive... I.M. Lee et al., "Effect of Physical Inactivity on Major Non-communicable Diseases Worldwide: An Analysis of Burden on Disease and Life Expectancy," *The Lancet* 380(9838), 21 July 2012, pp. 219–229.

Insufficient sleep... M. St-Onge et al., "Sleep Duration and Quality: Impact on Lifestyle Behaviors and Cardiometabolic Health: A Scientific Statement from the American Heart Association," *Circulation* 134(18), 19 September 2016, pp. e367–e386.

These are likely... E. Tobaldini et al., "Effects of Acute and Chronic Sleep Deprivation on Cardiovascular Regulation," *Archives Italiennes de Biologie* 152(2–3), 1 June 2014, pp. 103–110.

Sleep researchers... M. Hirshkowitz et al., "National Sleep Foundation's Updated Sleep Duration Recommendations: Final Report," *Sleep Health* 1(4), 1 December 2015, pp. 233–243.

These are all strongly... M.A. Whooley and J.M. Wong, "Depression and Cardiovascular Disorders," *Annual Review of Clinical Psychology* 9, 2013, pp. 327–354 and A.M. Roest et al., "Anxiety and Risk of Incident Coronary Heart Disease: A Meta-analysis," *Journal of the American College of Cardiology* 56(1), 29 June 2010, pp. 38–46 and Y. Chida and A. Steptoe, "The Association of Anger and Hostility with Future Coronary Heart Disease: A Meta-analytic Review of Prospective Evidence," *Journal of the American College of Cardiology* 53(11), 17 March 2009, pp. 936–946.

Loneliness and isolation... C.M. Perissinotto et al., "Loneliness in Older Persons: A Predictor of Functional Decline and Death," *Archives of Internal Medicine* 172, 23 July 2012, pp. 1,078–1,083.

Over time... P.H. Wirtz and R. von Känel, "Psychological Stress, Inflammation, and Coronary Heart Disease," *Current Cardiology Reports* 19(11), 20 September 2017, p. 111 and N. Glozier et al., "Psychosocial Risk Factors for Coronary Heart Disease," *Medical Journal*

of Australia 199(3), 2013, pp. 179–180.

Chapter 2

Harvard researchers... Y. Li et al., "Impact of Healthy Lifestyle Factors on Life Expectancies in the US Population," *Circulation* 138(4), 30 April 2018, pp. 345–355.

As amazing... N. Mehta and M. Myrskylä, "The Population Health Benefits of a Healthy Lifestyle: Life Expectancy Increased and Onset of Disability Delayed," *Health Affairs* 36(8), August 2017, pp. 1,495–1,502.

One study like... The Diabetes Prevention Program Research Group, "The Diabetes Prevention Program (DPP)," *Diabetes Care* 25(12), December 2002, pp. 2,165–2,171.

Studies looking at... M.Y. Johansen et al., "Effect of an Intensive Lifestyle Intervention on Glycemic Control in Patients with Type 2 Diabetes: A Randomized Clinical Trial," *Journal of the American Medical Association* 318(7), 15 August 2017, pp. 637–646.

In a study... M.E. Lean et al., "Primary Care-Led Weight Management for Remission of Type 2 Diabetes (DiRECT): An Open-Label, Cluster-Randomized

Trial," *The Lancet* 391(10120), 10 February 2018, pp. 541–551.

Cardiologist, researcher... L.G. Gilstrap et al., "Community-Based Primary Prevention Programs Decrease the Rate of Metabolic Syndrome among Socioeconomically Disadvantaged Women," *Journal of Women's Health* 22(4), April 2013, pp. 322–329.

It was many decades... D. Ornish et al., "Can Lifestyle Changes Reverse Coronary Heart Disease? The Lifestyle Heart Trial," *The Lancet* 336(8708), 21 July 1990, pp. 129–133.

One of his early... D. Ornish et al., "Intensive Lifestyle Changes for Reversal of Coronary Heart Disease," *Journal of the American Medical Association* 280(23), 16 December 1998, pp. 2001–2007.

The trial was so... D. Ornish, "Avoiding Revascularization with Lifestyle Changes: The Multicenter Lifestyle Demonstration Project," *The American Journal of Cardiology* 82(10B), 26 November 1998, pp. 72T–76T.

The program has been... A. Silberman et al., "The Effectiveness and Efficacy of an Intensive Cardiac Rehabilitation Program in 24 Sites," *American Journal of Health Promotion* 24(4), March–April 2010, pp. 260–266

and W. Zeng et al., "Benefits and Costs of Intensive Lifestyle Modification Programs for Symptomatic Coronary Disease in Medicare Beneficiaries," *American Heart Journal* 165(5), May 2013, pp. 785–792.

One recent study compared... R.A. Carels et al., "A Randomized Trial Comparing Two Approaches to Weight Loss: Differences in Weight Loss Maintenance," *Journal of Health Psychology* 19(2), February 2014, pp. 296–311.

Another study of five hundred and twenty obese... R.J. Beeken et al., "Study Protocol for the Ten Top Tips (10TT) Trial: A Randomized Controlled Trial of Habit-Based Advice for Weight Control in General Practice," *BMC Public Health* 12, 16 August 2012, p. 667 and R.J. Beeken et al., "A Brief Intervention for Weight Control Based on Habit-Formation Theory Delivered Through Primary Care: Results from a Randomized Controlled Trial," *International Journal of Obesity* 41(2), 2017, pp. 246–254.

What were those ten... Supplementary material to R.J. Beeken et al., 2017.

In a follow-up... "The 'Power' to Trade Naughty Habits for Nice Ones," NPR *Talk of the Nation*, 24 December 2012, www.npr .org/2012/12/24/167977418/

the-power-to-trade-naughty-habits-for-nice-ones.

Studies show (social support)... A. Compare et al., "Social Support, Depression, and Heart Disease: A Ten Year Literature Review," *Frontiers in Psychology* 4, 1 July 2013, p. 384.

Studies show (plant-based diet)... D. Aune et al., "Fruit and Vegetable Intake and the Risk of Cardiovascular Disease, Total Cancer, and All-Cause Mortality: A Systematic Review and Dose-Response Meta-analysis of Prospective Studies," *International Journal of Epidemiology* 46(3), 1 June 2017, pp. 1,029–1,056.

It's true that (alcohol)... B. Xi et al., "Relationship of Alcohol Consumption to All-Cause, Cardiovascular, and Cancer-Related Mortality in US Adults," *Journal of the American College of Cardiology* 70(8), 22 August 2017, pp. 913–922.

Chapter 3

In a 2013 survey... N.B. Anderson et al., "Stress in America," American Psychological Association, 11 February 2014, www.apa.org/news/press/releases/stress/2013/stress-report.pdf.

What can make... P. Björntorp, "Do Stress Reactions Cause Abdominal Obesity and

Comorbidities?," *Obesity Reviews: An Official Journal of the International Association for the Study of Obesity* 2(2), May 2001, pp. 73–86.

Change Your Identity... N. Eyal, "Can't Kick a Bad Habit? You're Probably Doing It Wrong," *Psychology Today*, posted 3 April 2015, www.psychologytoday.com/us/blog/automatic-you/201504/can-t-kick-bad-habit-you-re-probably-doing-it-wrong and N. Eyal, "The Behavioral Economics Diet: The Science of Killing a Bad Habit," *Nir and Far*, www.nirandfar.com/2015/05/behavioral-economics-diet-the-science-of-killing-a-bad-habit .html. Accessed May 2018.

Researchers trying to... P. Lally et al., "How Are Habits Formed: Modeling Habit Information in the Real World," *European Journal of Social Psychology* 40, 2010, pp. 998–1,009.

Chapter 4

Several studies have... M.R. Montinari et al., "History of Music Therapy and Its Contemporary Applications in Cardiovascular Diseases," *Southern Medical Journal* 111(2), 1 February 2018, pp. 98–102.

In a 2015 Italian study... L. Gruhlke et al., "Mozart, But Not the Beatles, Reduces Systolic

Blood Pressure in Patients with Myocardial Infarction," *Acta Cardiologia* 70(6), 1 June 2015, pp. 703–706.

In a 2016 German study... H. Trappe and G. Voit, "The Cardiovascular Effect of Musical Genres," *Deutsches Ärzteblatt International* 113(20), 20 May 2016, pp. 347–352.

Herbert Benson, MD, conducted... H. Benson, "The Relaxation Response: History, Physiological Basis, and Clinical Usefulness," *Acta Medica Scandinavica. Supplementum* 660, 1982, pp. 231–237.

Positive emotions... N.L. Sin, "The Protective Role of Positive Well-Being in Cardiovascular Disease: Review of Current Evidence, Mechanisms, and Clinical Implications," *Current Cardiology Reports* 18(11), November 2016, p. 106.

One 2011 English study... J.K. Boehm et al., "A Prospective Study of Positive Psychological Well-Being and Coronary Heart Disease," *Health Psychology: Official Journal of the Division of Health Psychology, American Psychological Association* 30(3), May 2011, pp. 259–267.

Other studies show (positive emotions)... C.M. DuBois et al., "Positive Psychological Attributes and Cardiac Outcomes:

Associations, Mechanisms, and Interventions," *Psychosomatics* 53(4), 2012, pp. 303–318.

In one fun study... T.L. Kraft and S.D. Pressman, "Grin and Bear It: The Influence of Manipulated Facial Expression on the Stress Response," *Psychological Science* 23(11), 2012, pp. 1,372–1,378.

Multiple research studies (exercise)... M.E. Hopkins et al., "Differential Effects of Acute and Regular Physical Exercise on Cognition and Affect," *Neuroscience* 215, 26 July 2012, pp. 59–68 and I.H. Jonsdottir et al., "A Prospective Study of Leisure-Time Physical Activity and Mental Health in Swedish Health Care Workers and Social Insurance Officers," *Preventive Medicine* 51(5), November 2010, pp. 373–377 and A.C. King et al., "Effects of Moderate-Intensity Exercise on Physiological, Behavioral, and Emotional Responses to Family Caregiving: A Randomized Controlled Trial," *The Journals of Gerontology. Series A, Biological Sciences and Medical Sciences* 57(1), January 2002, pp. M26–36.

Plenty of observational... C.E. Jenkinson et al., "Is Volunteering a Public Health Intervention? A Systematic Review and Meta-analysis of the Health and Survival of Volunteers," *BMC Public Health* 23, August 2013, p. 773.

In a study of three hundred and forty adults... S.H. Han et al., "Stress-Buffering Effects of Volunteering on Salivary Cortisol: Results from a Daily Diary Study," *Social Science and Medicine* 201, March 2018, pp. 120–126.

In one study, researchers (gratitude)... R.A. Emmons and M.E. McCullough, "Counting Blessings Versus Burdens: An Experimental Investigation of Gratitude and Subjective Well-Being in Daily Life," *Journal of Personality and Social Psychology* 84, February 2003, pp. 377–389.

Another study applied... L.S. Redwine et al., "Pilot Randomized Study of a Gratitude Journaling Intervention on Heart Rate Variability and Inflammatory Biomarkers in Patients with Stage B Heart Failure," *Psychosomatic Medicine* 78(6), July–August 2016, pp. 667–676.

Making a daily habit... A.M. Wood et al., "Gratitude and Well-Being: A Review and Theoretical Integration," *Clinical Psychology Review* 30(7), November 2010, pp. 890–905.

A 2016 analysis... M. Soga et al., "Gardening Is Beneficial for Health: A Meta-analysis," *Preventive Medicine Reports* 5, online, 14 November 2016, pp. 92–99.

There is scientific evidence that these negative emotions... J.M. Wong et al., "Hostility, Health Behaviors, and Risk of Recurrent Events in Patients with Stable Coronary Heart Disease: Findings from the Heart and Soul Study," *Journal of the American Heart Association* 2(5), 30 September 2013, p.e000052 and M. McCullough et al., "Vengefulness: Relationships with Forgiveness, Rumination, Well-Being, and the Big Five," *Personality and Social Psychology Bulletin* 27(5), 1 May 2001, pp. 601–610.

It follows, of course... S. Menaham and M. Love, "Forgiveness in Psychotherapy: The Key to Healing," *Journal of Clinical Psychology* 69(8), August 2013, pp. 829–835.

Forgiveness, including... D.J. Kearney et al., "Loving-Kindness Meditation for Post-traumatic Stress Disorder: A Pilot Study," *Journal of Traumatic Stress* 26(4), August 2013, pp. 426–434.

The human-animal bond... E. Friedmann and H. Son, "The Human-Companion Animal Bond: How Humans Benefit," *The Veterinary Clinics of North America. Small Animal Practice* 39(2), March 2009, pp. 293–326.

Animal-assisted therapy... L.S. Muñoz et al., "Animal-Assisted Interventions in Internal and Rehabilitation Medicine: A Review of the Recent Literature," *Panminerva Medica* 53(2), June 2011, pp. 129–136.

But you can experience... S. Feldman, "Alleviating Anxiety, Stress, and Depression with the Pet Effect," Anxiety and Depression Association of America, https://adaa.org/learn-from-us/from-the-experts/blog-posts/consumer/alleviating-anxiety-stress-and-depression-pet. Accessed May 2018.

In one recent study... A. Ewert and Y. Chang, "Levels of Nature and Stress Response," *Behavioral Sciences* (Basel) 8(5), 17 May 2018, pii. E49.

Moderate-pressure massage... T. Field, "Massage Therapy Research Review," *Complementary Therapies in Clinical Practice* 20(4), November 2014, pp. 224–229 and M.A. Diego et al., "Massage Therapy of Moderate and Light Pressure and Vibrator Effects on EEG and Heart Rate," *The International Journal of Neuroscience* 114(1), January 2004, pp. 31–44 and M. Hernandez-Reif et al., "High Blood Pressure and Associated Symptoms Were Reduced by Massage Therapy," *Journal of Bodywork and Movement Therapies* 4(1), January 2000, pp. 31–38 and S.M. Kubsch, T. Neveau, and K. Vandertie, "Effect of Cutaneous Stimulation on Pain Reduction in Emergency Department Patients," *Complementary Therapies in Nursing and Midwifery* 6(1), February 2000, pp. 25–32 and M.S. Kim et al., "Effects of Hand Massage on Anxiety in Cataract Surgery Patients Using Local Anesthesia," *Journal of Cataract and Refractive Surgery* 27(6), June 2001, pp. 884–890.

The National Center for Complementary and Integrative Health... Fact Sheet on Massage. https://nccih.nih.gov/health/massage/massageintroduction.htm.

These amazing molecules... R.M. Bruno and L. Ghiadoni, "Polyphenols, Antioxidants, and the Sympathetic Nervous System," *Current Pharmaceutical Design* 24 (2), 2018, pp. 130–139.

Sleep deprivation... E. Tobaldini et al., "Effects of Acute and Chronic Sleep Deprivation on Cardiovascular Regulation," *Archives Italiennes de Biologie* 152(2–3), 1 June 2014, pp. 103–110.

One of the first... and *The blue light (sleep)...* A. Qaseem, "Management of Chronic Insomnia Disorder in Adults: A Clinical Practice Guideline from the American College of Physicians," *Annals of Internal Medicine* 165(2), 19 July 2016, pp. 125–133 and E. Zhou, "Sleep

Problems: The Most Effective Lifestyle Medicine Interventions," Lecture, Lifestyle Medicine: Tools for Promoting Healthy Change Course of Harvard Medical School, 23 June 2018.

Studies show… and When families eat… J.B. de Wit et al., "Food Culture in the Home Environment: Family Meal Practices and Values Can Support Healthy Eating and Self-Regulation in Young People in Four European Countries," *Applied Psychology: Health and Well-Being* 7(1), March 2015, pp. 22–40.

When elderly people… Y. Kimura et al., "Eating Alone among Community-Dwelling Japanese Elderly: Association with Depression and Food Diversity," *The Journal of Nutrition, Health, and Aging* 16(8), August 2012, pp. 728–731.

Overall, people who… J.A. Fulkerson et al., "A Review of Associations Between Family or Shared Meal Frequency and Dietary and Weight Status Outcomes Across the Lifespan," *Journal of Nutrition Education and Behavior* 46(1), January 2014, pp. 2–19.

Studies show that… and People can feel lonely… S. Cacioppo et al., "Toward a Neurology of Loneliness," *Psychological Bulletin*

140(6), November 2014, pp. 1,464–1,504.

Chapter 5

There are mountains of… "The Nutrition Source: Fruits and Vegetables," Harvard T.H. Chan School of Public Health, www.hsph.harvard.edu/ nutritionsource/what-should-you-eat/vegetables-and-fruits/. Accessed May 2018 and M. de Lorgeril et al., "Mediterranean Diet, Traditional Risk Factors, and the Rate of Cardiovascular Complications after Myocardial Infarction: Final Report of the Lyon Diet Heart Study," *Circulation* 99(6), 16 February 1999, pp. 779–785 and K.R. Tuttle et al., "Comparison of Low-Fat Versus Mediterranean-Style Dietary Intervention after First Myocardial Infarction," *The American Journal of Cardiology* 101(11), 1 June 2008, pp. 1,523–1,530.

An analysis of almost one hundred… D. Aune et al., "Fruit and Vegetable Intake and the Risk of Cardiovascular Disease, Total Cancer, and All-Cause Mortality: A Systematic Review and Dose-Response Meta-analysis of Prospective Studies," *International Journal of Epidemiology* 46(3), 1 June 2017, pp. 1,029–1,056.

These contain natural… J. Hever, "Plant-Based Diets: A Physician's

Guide," *The Permanente Journal* 20(3), Summer 2016, pp. 93–101.

Studies have shown… L. Blekkenhorst et al., "Cruciferous and Total Vegetable Intakes Are Inversely Associated with Subclinical Atherosclerosis in Older Adult Women," *Journal of the American Heart Association* 7(8), 4 April 2018, p. e008391 and R. Pollock, "The Effect of Green Leafy and Cruciferous Vegetable Intake on the Incidence of Cardiovascular Disease: A Meta-analysis," *JRSM Cardiovascular Disease* 5, December 2016, pp 1–9.

Going overboard… W.J. Choi and J. Kim, "Dietary Factors and the Risk of Thyroid Cancer: A Review," *Clinical Nutrition Research* 3(2), July 2014, pp. 75–88.

The American Heart Association… L. Horn et al., "Recommended Dietary Pattern to Achieve Adherence to the American Heart Association/American College of Cardiology (AHA/ ACC) Guidelines," *Circulation* 134(22), 29 November 2016, pp. e505–e529.

Dietary fiber… "The Nutrition Source: Fiber," Harvard T.H. Chan School of Public Health, www.hsph.harvard.edu/ nutritionsource/carbohydrates/ fiber/ and "Dietary Fiber," US

Department of Health and Human Services/Federal Drug Administration, www.accessdata.fda.gov/scripts/interactivenutritionfactslabel/factsheets/dietary_fiber.pdf. Accessed May 2018.

A cup of cooked garbanzo... T. Wallace et al., "The Nutritional Value and Health Benefits of Chickpeas and Hummus," *Nutrients* 8(12), December 2016, p. 766.

People who eat legumes... I. Abete et al., "Obesity and the Metabolic Syndrome: Role of Different Dietary Macronutrient Distribution Patterns and Specific Nutritional Components on Weight Loss and Maintenance," *Nutrition Reviews* 68(4), April 2010, pp. 214–231 and C.J. Rebello et al., "A Review of the Nutritional Value of Legumes and Their Effects on Obesity and Its Related Co-morbidities," *Obesity Reviews: An Official Journal of the International Association for the Study of Obesity* 15(5), May 2014, pp. 392–407.

Regular intake (PUFAs)... "Omega-3 Fatty Acids," National Institutes of Health Office of Dietary Supplements, updated 6 June 2018, https://ods.od.nih.gov/factsheets/omega3fattyacids-healthprofessional/.

There has been some controversy... M. Bittman, "Butter Is Back," *The New York Times*, posted 25 March 2014, www.nytimes.com/2014/03/26/opinion/bittman-butter-is-back.html and A. Sifferlin, "The Case for Eating Butter Just Got Stronger," *Time*, posted 29 June 2016, http://time.com/4386248/fat-butter-nutrition-health/.

citing studies that showed no... R. Chowdhury et al., "Association of Dietary, Circulating, and Supplement Fatty Acids with Coronary Risk: A Systematic Review and Meta-analysis," *Annals of Internal Medicine* 160(6), 18 March 2014, pp. 398–406 and L. Pimpin et al., "Is Butter Back? A Systematic Review and Meta-analysis of Butter Consumption and Risk of Cardiovascular Disease, Diabetes, and Total Mortality," *PLoS One* 11(6), 29 June 2016, p. e0158118.

The science community... B. Moran, "Is Butter Really Back?," *Harvard Public Health* magazine, www.hsph.harvard.edu/magazine/magazine_article/is-butter-really-back/ and "The Nutrition Source: We Repeat, Butter Is Not Back," Harvard T.H. Chan School of Public Health, posted 30 June 2016, www.hsph.harvard.edu/nutritionsource/2016/06/30/we-repeat-butter-is-not-back/.

hitting back with headlines like... M. Nestle, "No, Butter Is Not Back (Eat in Moderation, Please)," *Food Politics Blog*, posted 6 July 2016, www.foodpolitics.com/2016/07/no-butter-is-not-back-eat-in-moderation-please.

Research backs... Y. Li, "Saturated Fats Compared with Unsaturated Fats and Sources of Carbohydrates in Relation to Risk of Coronary Heart Disease: A Prospective Cohort Study," *Journal of the American College of Cardiology* 66(14), 6 October 2015, pp. 1,538–1,548.

When we directly compare... D. Mozaffarian et al., "Effects on Coronary Heart Disease of Increasing Polyunsaturated Fat in Place of Saturated Fat: A Systematic Review and Meta-analysis of Randomized Controlled Trials," *PLoS Medicine* 7(3), March 2010, p. e1000252 and L. Hooper et al., "Reduction in Saturated Fat Intake for Cardiovascular Disease," *The Cochrane Database of Systematic Reviews* (6), 10 June 2015, CD011737.

Another study... R. Estruch et al., "Primary Prevention of Cardiovascular Disease with a Mediterranean Diet," *New England Journal of Medicine* 368, 4 April 2013, pp. 1,279–1,290; (retraction and republication: *New England Journal of Medicine* 378(25), 21 June 2018, p. e34).

if we replace the less-healthy... F. Sacks et al., "Dietary Fats and Cardiovascular Disease: A Presidential Advisory from the American Heart Association," *Circulation* 136(3), 15 June 2017, pp. e1–e23.

Research shows that (nuts)... A.J. Mayhew et al.: "A Systematic Review and Meta-analysis of Nut Consumption and Incident Risk of CVD and All-Cause Mortality," *The British Journal of Nutrition* 115(2), 28 January 2016, pp. 212–225.

Another study found... Y.Q. Weng et al., "Association Between Nut Consumption and Coronary Heart Disease: A Meta-analysis," *Coronary Artery Disease* 27(3), May 2016, pp. 227–232.

Research has consistently... E. Higginbotham and P.R. Taub, "Cardiovascular Benefits of Dark Chocolate?," *Current Treatment Options in Cardiovascular Medicine* 17(12), December 2015, p. 54 and S. Yuan et al., "Chocolate Consumption and Risk of Coronary Heart Disease, Stroke, and Diabetes: A Meta-analysis of Prospective Studies," *Nutrients* 9(7), 2017, p. 688 and C.S. Kwok et al., "Habitual Chocolate Consumption and Risk of Cardiovascular Disease among Healthy Men and Women," *Heart* 101(16), August 2015, pp. 1,279–1,287.

Herbs (parts of leafy)... M. Aggarwal et al., "Integrative

Medicine for Cardiovascular Disease and Prevention," *Medical Clinics of North America* 101(5), September 2017, pp. 895–923 and K. Griffiths et al., "Food Antioxidants and Their Anti-inflammatory Properties: A Potential Role in Cardiovascular Diseases and Cancer Prevention," *Diseases* 4(3), 1 August 2016, p. 28 and M. Greger and G. Stone, *How Not to Die* (New York, NY: Flatiron Books, 2015) and S. Jiang et al., "Curcumin As a Potential Protective Compound Against Cardiac Diseases," *Pharmacological Research* 119, May 2017, pp. 373–383.

Extra herb and spice... Q. Li et al., "Enjoyment of Spicy Flavors Enhances Central Salty-Taste Perception and Reduces Salt Intake and Blood Pressure," *Hypertension* 70(6), December 2017, pp. 1,291–1,299.

There is ample... B.V. Reamy et al., "Prevention of Cardiovascular Disease," *Primary Care: Clinics in Office Practice* 45(1), 2018, pp. 25–44 and D. Aune et al., "Fruit and Vegetable Intake and the Risk of Cardiovascular Disease, Total Cancer, and All-Cause Mortality: A Systematic Review and Dose-Response Meta-analysis of Prospective Studies," *International Journal of Epidemiology* 46(3), 1 June 2017, pp. 1,029–1,056.

All animal-based products... M. Song et al., "Association

of Animal and Plant Protein Intake with All-Cause and Cause-Specific Mortality," *JAMA Internal Medicine* 176(10), 1 October 2016, pp. 1,453–1,463.

A high-sodium... S.S. Anand et al., "Food Consumption and Its Impact on Cardiovascular Disease: Importance of Solutions Focused on the Globalized Food System: A Report from the Workshop Convened by the World Heart," *Journal of the American College of Cardiology* 66(14), 6 October 2015, pp. 1,590–1,614.

Both green and black... M. Aggarwal et al., "Integrative Medicine for Cardiovascular Disease and Prevention," *Medical Clinics of North America* 101(5), September 2017, pp. 895–923.

For most people... J.H. O'Keefe et al., "Coffee for Cardioprotection and Longevity," *Progress in Cardiovascular Disease*, 21 February 2018 (epub) and A.M. Miranda et al., "Coffee Consumption and Coronary Artery Calcium Score: Cross-Sectional Results of ELSA-Brasil (Brazilian Longitudinal Study of Adult Health)," *Journal of the American Heart Association* 7(7), 3 April 2018, p. e007155 and R. Poole et al., "Coffee Consumption and Health: Umbrella Review of Meta-analyses of Multiple Health

Outcomes," *The BMJ* 359, 22 November 2017, p. j5024.

Research shows that... and *Drinking any amount (alcohol)...* S. Bell et al., "Association Between Clinically Recorded Alcohol Consumption and Initial Presentation of 12 Cardiovascular Diseases: Population Based Cohort Study Using Linked Health Records," *The BMJ* 356, 22 March 2017, p. j909 and P.E. Ronksley et al., "Association of Alcohol Consumption with Selected Cardiovascular Disease Outcomes: A Systematic Review and Meta-analysis," *The BMJ* 342, 22 February 2011, p. d671.

Alcohol can also... C. Tangney et al., "Cardiac Benefits and Risks ... UpToDate, updated March 2018, https://www.uptodate.com/contents/cardiovascular-benefits-and-risks-of-moderate-alcohol-consumption.

People who make their own... Reicks M et al, "Impact of Cooking and Home Food Preparation Interventions Among Adults: A Systematic Review," *Journal of Nutrition Education and Behavior* 50(2) February 2018, pp. 148–172.

There is a link (dental)... Harvard Health Letter, "Gum Disease and Heart Disease: The Common Thread," published March 2018, https://www.health.harvard.edu/heart-health/
gum-disease-and-heart-disease-the-common-thread.

Chapter 6

An analysis of fifty-four... C. Ma et al., "Effects of Weight Loss Interventions for Adults Who Are Obese on Mortality, Cardiovascular Disease, and Cancer: Systematic Review and Meta-analysis," *The BMJ* 359, 14 November 2017, p. j4849.

Scientific studies have... J.F. Guthrie et al., "Role of Food Prepared Away from Home in the American Diet, 1977–78 Versus 1994–96: Change and Consequences," *Journal of Nutrition Education and Behavior* 34(3), May–June 2002, pp. 140–150.

Many studies have shown... J.A. Fulkerson, "Away-from-Home Family Dinner Sources and Associations with Weight Status, Body Composition, and Related Biomarkers of Chronic Disease among Adolescents and Their Parents," *Journal of the American Dietetic Association* 111(12), December 2011, pp. 1,892–1,897.

A study of more than forty... P. Ducrot et al., "Meal Planning Is Associated with Food Variety, Diet Quality, and Body Weight Status in a Large Sample of French Adults," *International*

Journal of Behavioral Nutrition and Physical Activity 14(1), 2 February 2017, p.12.

A much-awaited... C.D. Gardner et al., "Effect of Low-Fat vs. Low-Carbohydrate Diet on 12-Month Weight Loss in Overweight Adults and the Association with Genotype Pattern or Insulin Secretion: The DIETFITS Randomized Clinical Trial," *Journal of the American Medical Association* 319(7), 20 February 2018, pp. 667–679; erratum in: *Journal of the American Medical Association* 319(13), 3 April 2018, p. 1,386 and *Journal of the American Medical Association* 319(16), 24 April 2018, p. 1,728.

Most studies (artificial sweeteners)... J.R. Roberts, "The Paradox of Artificial Sweeteners in Managing Obesity," *Current Gastroenterology Reports* 17(1), January 2015, p. 423.

One possible explanation... M.V. Burke and D.M. Small, "Physiological Mechanisms by Which Non-nutritive Sweeteners May Impact Body Weight and Metabolism," *Physiology and Behavior* 152(Pt B), 1 December 2015, pp. 381–388.

Research studies show (portion control)... and *People who have (routine)...* S. Ramage et al., "Healthy Strategies for Successful Weight Loss and Weight Maintenance: A Systematic

Review," *Applied Physiology, Nutrition, and Metabolism* 39(1), January 2014, pp. 1–20.

In a 2013 survey... N.B. Anderson et al., "Stress in America," American Psychological Association, 11 February 2014, www.apa.org/news/press/releases/stress/2013/stress-report.pdf.

Research suggests... S. Leow et al., "A Role for Exercise in Attenuating Unhealthy Food Consumption in Response to Stress," *Nutrients* 10(2), 6 February 2018, pii. E176.

Multiple studies (tracking food)... L.E. Burke et al., "Self-monitoring in Weight Loss: A Systematic Review of the Literature," *Journal of the American Dietetic Association* 111(1), January 2011, pp. 92–102.

In a study of (logging food)... S.L. Painter et al., "What Matters in Weight Loss? An In-Depth Analysis of Self-monitoring," *Journal of Medical Internet Research* 19(5), 12 May 2017, p. e160.

Studies show that (regular weighing)... D.M. Steinberg et al., "Weighing Every Day Matters: Daily Weighing Improves Weight Loss and Adoption of Weight Control Behaviors," *Journal of the Academy of Nutrition and Dietetics* 115(4), April 2015, pp. 511–518.

Note: studies show that colorful... I. Abete et al., "Obesity and the Metabolic Syndrome: Role of Different Dietary Macronutrient Distribution Patterns and Specific Nutritional Components on Weight Loss and Maintenance," *Nutrition Reviews* 68(4), April 2010, pp. 214–231 and P.K. Newby et al., "Food Patterns Measured by Factor Analysis and Anthropometric Changes in Adults," *The American Journal of Clinical Nutrition* 80(2), 1 August 2004, pp. 504–513 and C.J. Rebello et al., "A Review of the Nutritional Value of Legumes and Their Effects on Obesity and Its Related Co-morbidities," *Obesity Reviews: An Official Journal of the International Association for the Study of Obesity* 15(5), May 2014, pp. 392–407.

A scientific review of... P. Clifton, "Assessing the Evidence for Weight Loss Strategies in People with and Without Type 2 Diabetes," *World Journal of Diabetes* 8(10), 15 October 2017, pp. 440–454.

New studies suggest... J.F. Trepanowski et al., "Effect of Alternate-Day Fasting on Weight Loss, Weight Maintenance, and Cardioprotection among Metabolically Healthy Obese Adults," *JAMA Internal Medicine* 177(7), July 2017, pp. 930–938 and L.K. Heilbronn et al., "Alternate-Day Fasting in Nonobese Subjects: Effects on Body Weight, Body Composition, and Energy Metabolism," *The American Journal of Clinical Nutrition* 81(1), 1 January 2005, pp. 69–73 and L. Harris et al., "Intermittent Fasting Interventions for Treatment of Overweight and Obesity in Adults: A Systematic Review and Meta-analysis," *JBI Database of Systematic Reviews and Implementation Reports* 16(2), February 2018, pp. 507–547.

In one study... E.F. Sutton et al., "Early Time-Restricted Feeding Improves Insulin Sensitivity, Blood Pressure, and Oxidative Stress Even Without Weight Loss in Men with Prediabetes," *Cell Metabolism* 27(6), 5 June 2018, pp. 1,212–1,221.

Studies like this... R. Patterson and D. Sears, "Metabolic Effects of Intermittent Fasting," *Annual Review of Nutrition* 37, August 2017, pp. 371–393.

Research shows that... Fatima Cody Stanford, Harvard.edu Media Gallery, https://scholar.harvard.edu/fatimacodystanford/media-gallery/detail/159116/664186. Accessed May 2018.

She emphasizes... D.K. Patel and F.C. Stanford, "Safety and Tolerability of New-Generation

Anti-obesity Medications: A Narrative Review," *Postgraduate Medicine* 130(2), March 2018, pp. 173–182.

Research shows that (obesity medications)... T.K. Kyle and F.C. Stanford, "Low Utilization of Obesity Medications: What Are the Implications for Clinical Care?," *Obesity* (Silver Spring) 24(9), September 2016, p. 1,832.

Chapter 7

In a 2014 analysis (running)... D. Lee et al., "Leisure-Time Running Reduces All-Cause and Cardiovascular Mortality Risk," *Journal of the American College of Cardiology* 64(5), August 2014, pp. 472–481.

One analysis looking (sitting)... J.Y. Chau et al., "Daily Sitting Time and All-Cause Mortality: A Meta-analysis," *PLoS One* 8(11), 13 November 2013, p. e80000.

another study showed... S.S. Thosar et al., "Effect of Prolonged Sitting and Breaks in Sitting Time on Endothelial Function," *Medicine and Science in Sports and Exercise* 47(4), April 2015, pp. 843–849.

In a 2017 (housework)... S. Lear et al., "The Effect of Physical Activity on Mortality and Cardiovascular Disease in 130,000 People from 17

High-Income, Middle-Income, and Low-Income Countries: the PURE Study," *The Lancet* 390(10113), 16 December 2017, pp. 2,643–2,654.

In an analysis (activity monitors)... H.J. de Vries et al., "Do Activity Monitors Increase Physical Activity in Adults with Overweight or Obesity? A Systematic Review and Meta-analysis," *Obesity* (Silver Spring) 24(10), October 2016, pp. 2,078–2,091.

In another research study... S.L. Painter et al., "What Matters in Weight Loss? An In-Depth Analysis of Self-monitoring," *Journal of Medical Internet Research* 19(5), 12 May 2017, p. e160.

Studies show that (exercising with others)... S. Kanamori et al., "Exercising Alone Versus with Others and Associations with Subjective Health Status in Older Japanese: The JAGES Cohort Study," *Scientific Reports* 6, 15 December 2016, p. 39,151.

Researchers analyzed data and *TV sitting time is associated...* U. Ekelund et al., "Does Physical Activity Attenuate, Or Even Eliminate, the Detrimental Association of Sitting Time with Mortality? A Harmonized Meta-analysis of Data from More than One Million Men and Women," *The Lancet* 388(10051),

24 September 2016, pp. 1,302–1,310.

Chapter 8

Habit is defined... Definition of *Habit, Merriam-Webster Dictionary* online, updated on 8 August 2018, www.merriam-webster.com/dictionary/habit.

Addiction is defined... American Psychiatric Association. *The Diagnostic and Statistical Manual of Mental Disorders DSM-5.* (American Psychiatric Publishing, 2013).

Smokers die an... "The Health Consequences of Smoking—50 Years of Progress: A Report of the Surgeon General," Surgeon General website, www .surgeongeneral.gov/library/ reports/50-years-of-progress/fact-sheet.html. Accessed May 2018.

Heart health benefits... T. Takami and Y.-Saito, "Effects of Smoking Cessation on Central Blood Pressure and Arterial Stiffness," *Vascular Health and Risk Management* 7, 20 October 2011, pp. 633–638.

after a number of years, the risk... M. Shields and K. Wilkins, "Smoking, Smoking Cessation, and Heart Disease Risk: A 16-Year Follow-Up Study," *Health Reports* 24(2), February 2013, pp. 12–22.

Having a good quit plan... Y.K. Bartlett et al., "Effective Behavior Change Techniques in Smoking Cessation Interventions for People with Chronic Obstructive Pulmonary Disease: A Meta-analysis," *British Journal of Health Psychology* 19(1), February 2014, pp. 181–203.

In the US... "Economic Trends in Tobacco," The Centers for Disease Control and Prevention, updated 4 May 2018, www.cdc.gov/ tobacco/data_statistics/fact_sheets/ economics/econ_facts/index.htm.

In a study (stress eating)... T.Y. Pontes et al., "A Strategy for Weight Loss Based on Healthy Dietary Habits and Control of Eating Food," *Nutrición Hospitalaria* 31(6), 1 June 2015, pp. 2,392–2,399.

Binge eating disorder... F. Amianto et al., "Binge-Eating Disorder Diagnosis and Treatment: A Recap in Front of DSM-5," *BMC Psychiatry* 15:70, 3 April 2015.

You may have seen... N. Davis, "Is Sugar Really As Addictive As Cocaine? Scientists Row over Effect on Body and Brain," *The Guardian*, posted 25 August 2017, www.theguardian .com/society/2017/aug/25/ is-sugar-really-as-addictive-as-cocaine-scientists-row-over-effect-on-body-and-brain and T. Mann, "No, Sugar Isn't the New Heroin," posted 15 June 2017,

http://behavioralscientist.org/ no-sugar-isnt-new-heroin/.

Regardless of how... A. Carter et al., "The Neurobiology of 'Food Addiction' and Its Implications for Obesity Treatment and Policy," *Annual Review of Nutrition* 36, 17 July 2016, pp. 105–128.

Electronics use can... D.J. Kuss et al., "Internet Addiction: A Systematic Review of Epidemiological Research for the Last Decade," *Current Pharmaceutical Design* 20(25), 2014, pp. 4,026–4,052.

In a 2017 UK survey... "UK Public Are 'Glued to Smartphones' As Device Adoption Reaches New Heights," Deloitte Press Release, posted 20 September 2017, www2.deloitte .com/uk/en/pages/press-releases/ articles/uk-public-glued-to-smartphones.html.

A recent article... S. Dredge, "Mobile Phone Addiction? It's Time to Take Back Control," *The Guardian*, posted 27 January 2018, www.theguardian.com/ technology/2018/jan/27/mobile-phone-addiction-apps-break-the-habit-take-back-control.

Appendix C

US/Metric Conversion Chart

VOLUME CONVERSIONS	
US Volume Measure	Metric Equivalent
⅛ teaspoon	0.5 milliliter
¼ teaspoon	1 milliliter
½ teaspoon	2 milliliters
1 teaspoon	5 milliliters
½ tablespoon	7 milliliters
1 tablespoon (3 teaspoons)	15 milliliters
2 tablespoons (1 fluid ounce)	30 milliliters
¼ cup (4 tablespoons)	60 milliliters
⅓ cup	80 milliliters
½ cup (4 fluid ounces)	125 milliliters
⅔ cup	160 milliliters
¾ cup (6 fluid ounces)	180 milliliters
1 cup (16 tablespoons)	250 milliliters
1 pint (2 cups)	500 milliliters
1 quart (4 cups)	1 liter (about)

WEIGHT CONVERSIONS	
US Weight Measure	Metric Equivalent
½ ounce	15 grams
1 ounce	30 grams
2 ounces	60 grams
3 ounces	85 grams
¼ pound (4 ounces)	115 grams
½ pound (8 ounces)	225 grams
¾ pound (12 ounces)	340 grams
1 pound (16 ounces)	454 grams

OVEN TEMPERATURE CONVERSIONS	
Degrees Fahrenheit	Degrees Celsius
200 degrees F	95 degrees C
250 degrees F	120 degrees C
275 degrees F	135 degrees C
300 degrees F	150 degrees C
325 degrees F	160 degrees C
350 degrees F	180 degrees C
375 degrees F	190 degrees C
400 degrees F	205 degrees C
425 degrees F	220 degrees C
450 degrees F	230 degrees C

BAKING PAN SIZES	
American	Metric
8 × 1½ inch round baking pan	20 × 4 cm cake tin
9 × 1½ inch round baking pan	23 × 3.5 cm cake tin
11 × 7 × 1½ inch baking pan	28 × 18 × 4 cm baking tin
13 × 9 × 2 inch baking pan	30 × 20 × 5 cm baking tin
2 quart rectangular baking dish	30 × 20 × 3 cm baking tin
15 × 10 × 2 inch baking pan	38 × 25 × 5 cm baking tin (Swiss roll tin)
9 inch pie plate	22 × 4 or 23 × 4 cm pie plate
7 or 8 inch springform pan	18 or 20 cm springform or loose bottom cake tin
9 × 5 × 3 inch loaf pan	23 × 13 × 7 cm or 2 lb narrow loaf or pâté tin
1½ quart casserole	1.5 liter casserole
2 quart casserole	2 liter casserole

Index